The Caregiver's Guide
to Stroke Recovery

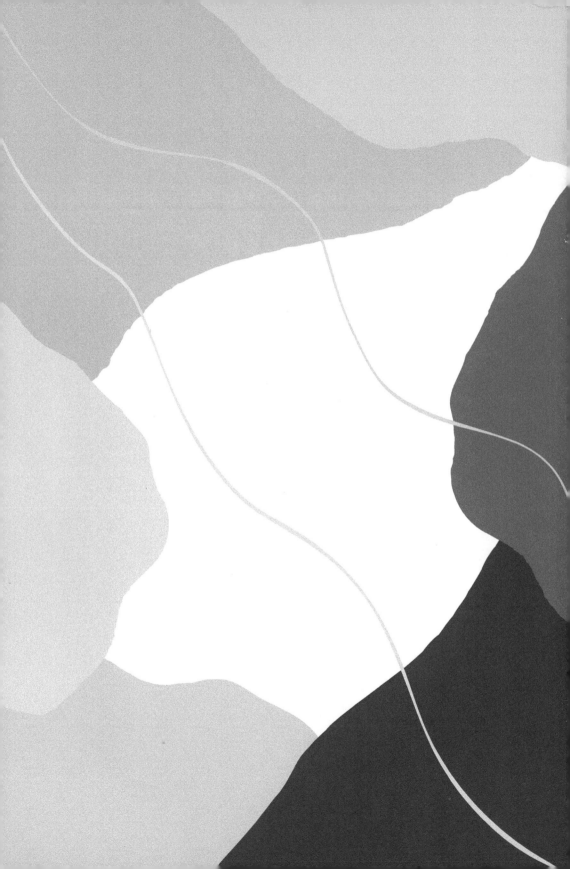

The CAREGIVER'S GUIDE to STROKE RECOVERY

Practical Advice for Caring for You and Your Loved One

Lucille Jorgensen, RN

ROCKRIDGE PRESS

Interior and Cover Designer: Lindsey Dekker
Art Producer: Tom Hood
Editor: Jed Bickman
Production Editor: Jenna Dutton
Production Manager: Michael Kay

Cover and interior illustrations courtesy Viktoria Lange/iStock; author photograph courtesy Michael Leone.

ISBN: Print 978-1-64876-577-3 | eBook 978-1-64876-578-0
R0

To my Lola, who is always an inspiration
and
To Auntie Lumen, whose light shines brightest

CONTENTS

INTRODUCTION

As a caregiver for a stroke survivor, you are on a remarkable journey that is both challenging and fulfilling. What you do is not easy, and I am happy that you're here. You and your loved one have embarked on a new stage in life, and it is my pleasure to be able to support and guide you.

I've been a nurse for almost 18 years, and I've worked in various healthcare fields such as telemetry, intensive care, cardiac catheterization, quality management, and acute rehabilitation. For the last few years, I've worked as the stroke program coordinator for a large academic hospital. I have found a new passion for working with stroke survivors, caregivers, and the healthcare team that supports them. The best part of my job is watching stroke patients and their caregivers grow together on the road to recovery.

Caregiving is a tough job, no matter what condition your loved one is in. It is incredibly rewarding, yet also one of the most tiring and emotionally draining jobs in the world. A caregiver's responsibilities are many, and I hope I can help by deepening your understanding of stroke and helping you make good decisions for yourself and your loved one.

In this book, you'll find chapters grouped into three major topics. First, I'll help you understand stroke and its impact on you and your loved one. The second section will discuss how to care for someone recovering from a stroke. Finally, I'll talk about you as a caregiver and the importance of self-care. I'm not going to let you forget about taking care of yourself, which is just as critical as taking care of your loved one.

In every chapter, you'll also find advice on what to do, what to say, and what to ask your healthcare team. My hope is that you will use these tips to become the best advocate for your loved one. The guidance provided in this book is meant to promote stroke recovery and provide vital caregiver support. And because taking care of yourself is so important, at the end of each chapter, I'll check in on you and see how you are doing. I'll ask you to examine how you're feeling and give you some advice on self-care.

The path to recovery lies in the partnership between stroke survivor and caregiver. The two of you are a team. All the laughter and the triumphs, the tears and frustration, create memories that will imprint on the soul. As partners, you and your loved one will share an enduring bond.

I wish you and your loved one the best. My deepest hope is that you find the advice in this book valuable and it truly helps you on your path together. Thank you for allowing me to support you and your loved one on your journey.

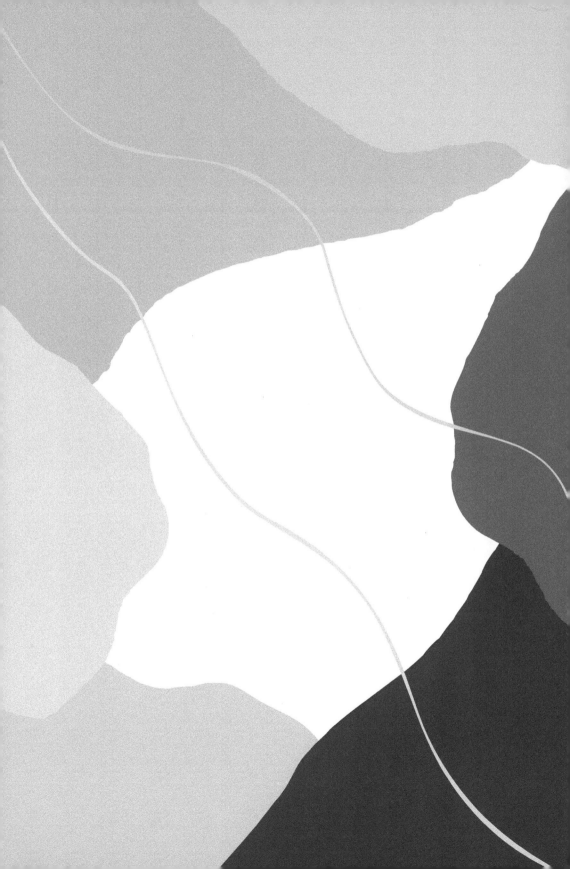

PART ONE

UNDERSTANDING STROKE

CHAPTER 1

STROKE EXPLAINED

Robin

Robin didn't know what to do. She sat by Rachel's hospital bed, holding her hand and listening to how scared her twin was. She could see how frustrated Rachel felt during her physical therapy. Robin did her best to put on a brave face for her sister, but she felt like crying inside. Truth was, she was scared and frustrated, too. She suspected Rachel knew this.

Four days ago, Rachel was over for their weekly family dinner. Robin and Rachel experienced everything together, and in 48 years, this hadn't changed. That is, until IT happened in the middle of dinner. Rachel's right arm suddenly went slack and crashed into her dinner plate, sending food flying. She was mumbling words, and the right side of her face looked like it was falling like melting wax. Robin was terrified—what was going on with her beloved sister? Robin's husband had the presence of mind to call 911.

Now in the hospital, Rachel could barely move her right leg and arm. She could speak better after the medication they gave her in the emergency room, and her face didn't look droopy, as it had before. But she would need to go to a rehab facility to regain the use of her right arm and leg strength. After that, she would live at Robin's house, and Robin would take care of her.

"Robin, I'm scared," Rachel said quietly.

"Me too," Robin confessed. "I don't know what to do. You and I will figure it out together. Partners in crime, remember?" She smiled at Rachel with tears in her eyes. "Who says we still can't laugh and grow old together?"

STROKE DEFINED

A stroke, or cerebrovascular accident (CVA), is a brain attack. A stroke occurs when the blood supply to a portion of the brain is cut off. The affected area loses its supply of oxygen, and the cells become damaged, or *ischemic*. Over time, this lack of oxygen will cause the cells to become permanently damaged or die, resulting in loss of brain function.

There are two types of stroke: ischemic strokes and hemorrhagic strokes. The brain requires a constant flow of blood, which delivers oxygen. Both types of stroke occur when the flow of blood and the oxygen it carries are disrupted. An ischemic stroke, the more common type, occurs when a blood clot causes a blockage in one of the brain's blood vessels. In hemorrhagic strokes, the blood supply may be disrupted when a weak part of the artery ruptures or breaks open and bleeding occurs within the brain tissue. In both types of stroke, brain cells die because they are cut off from their regular oxygen supply.

The most common misconception about stroke revolves around the urgency of seeking help. Most people delay getting help because they don't realize how serious strokes are. When someone is experiencing the signs and symptoms of a stroke, it is critical to call 911 immediately. Strokes are a medical emergency. For every minute that passes during a stroke, approximately two million brain cells die. In the healthcare field, there is a saying: "Time Is Brain." Rapid treatment is necessary to reduce the loss of function to the affected area of the brain. The best chance of recovery lies in getting emergency treatment as quickly as possible after the onset of initial symptoms. Delaying treatment can be devastating.

The brain is the control center of the body. It controls voluntary movements, such as walking and speaking, as well as involuntary functions, such as breathing and controlling digestion. Your brain houses your memories and emotions. It dictates your personality, who you are, and how you think and feel. The brain is responsible for processing all your senses, such as sight, smell, hearing, touch, and taste. It also regulates your ability to maintain your balance.

No two strokes are the same. Each person will experience different functional deficits depending on the stroke's location. The location of the stroke in the brain will determine the loss of function. Different parts of the brain are tasked with different functions. For example, each side of the brain controls movement and sensation on the body's opposite side. This is because of the way the nerves crisscross in the center of the brain. Someone suffering a stroke on the left side of their brain could experience the inability to move or feel their right arm or right leg.

If a stroke occurs in the front of the brain, there may be changes in behavior and mood. The person may undergo changes such as irritability, or impulsive or inappropriate behavior. They may also experience changes in their personality, such as frequent mood swings, apathy, or depression.

A stroke in the brain's speech centers can result in the inability to speak, called "aphasia." It can also result in difficulty speaking, such as slurring or garbling of words. Your loved one may struggle to find the right words to say (expressive aphasia) or have difficulty understanding what has been said to them (receptive aphasia). Aphasia is covered in greater depth in chapter 5.

Strokes can affect a person's ability to swallow (dysphagia) and can increase their risk of choking. Vision changes such as loss of peripheral vision, double vision, or blurred vision may occur when the stroke affects the back part of the brain, where the vision center is located. Stroke can also cause short- or long-term memory loss, which may interfere with the ability to function. Having a stroke puts a person at a higher risk of developing dementia than people who have not had a stroke. Approximately one in four people who have had a stroke will develop dementia.

The more severe the stroke, the more widespread the loss of function will be. As the brain cells die, the damage spreads, and more areas become affected. Mild loss of movement in the right hand may become permanent paralysis of the right hand and leg. What begins as mild slurring of words may progress to the inability to speak and swallow. This is why immediate medical attention is so critical. Major strokes, if left untreated, could lead to severe disability or even death. However, with proper treatment and rehabilitation, stroke survivors can regain lost function and make a meaningful recovery.

Ischemic Stroke

An ischemic stroke occurs when a blood vessel supplying blood and oxygen to the brain is narrowed or blocked. Have you ever left bacon grease in a pan? The grease hardens into a heavy, white sludge. High cholesterol levels (fat) in the blood can cause the same type of sludge to build up inside your arteries. Over time, the sludge hardens and becomes jagged, forming plaque. The rough edges of the plaque are perfect for catching platelets in the blood and forming a clot. If a clot gets large enough, it can completely block the artery. Also, little pieces of blood clots or plaque (called "emboli") can break off. These emboli flow downstream and get wedged in the brain's smaller vessels, further cutting off oxygen-carrying blood to the brain cells.

Transient Ischemic Attack (TIA)

Transient ischemic attacks, or TIAs, are also known as "mini-strokes." TIAs are caused by a temporary blockage to an artery of the brain that resolves on its own. TIAs do not cause any lasting damage but are considered to be an early warning sign of stroke. People who experience a TIA are at higher risk of a more severe stroke in the future.

Symptoms of a TIA are the same as a stroke. Symptoms come quickly and may last for a few seconds or even a few hours before resolving. If you are having symptoms of a stroke or TIA, call 911 and seek help right away. TIAs usually resolve within 24 hours, while stroke symptoms persist after 24 hours.

Cryptogenic Stroke

About 25 percent of ischemic strokes are classified as "cryptogenic." A cryptogenic stroke is a stroke of undetermined causes. This means the cause of the stroke can't be determined, despite extensive diagnostic testing.

Cryptogenic strokes are often associated with heart conditions such as atrial fibrillation or a patent foramen ovale. Atrial fibrillation is an irregular heart rhythm that causes the heart's upper chambers (atria) to beat out of sync with the bottom chambers of the heart (ventricles). In atrial fibrillation, the atria beat very quickly and agitate the blood, causing micro-clots. These clots float through the bloodstream and get lodged in the brain's smaller vessels, causing a stroke.

Having a patent foramen ovale can also increase the risk of micro-clots. The foramen ovale is a hole between the right and left atria that everyone has at birth. This hole often closes soon after birth. However, if the hole fails to close on its own, this is called "patent foramen ovale," and with this, micro-clots can form as blood flows between the atria. Micro-clots are not easily detectable through testing, so it's difficult to determine if they are the cause of a cryptogenic stroke.

Hemorrhagic Stroke

Hemorrhagic strokes are caused by a rupture in a blood vessel of the brain. Blood pours into the brain tissue, and nearby cells are cut off from their oxygen supply. As blood pools in the brain, it pushes the brain matter against the inside of the skull, causing more damage. Hemorrhagic strokes can be dangerous, as the brain's increasing pressure can cause the brain tissue to shift and become displaced.

The most common cause of hemorrhagic stroke is high blood pressure. Chronic high blood pressure puts a strain on the blood vessels and weakens their walls, causing them to split or break. Another cause of hemorrhagic stroke is a ruptured aneurysm. Aneurysms form when a weak part of the blood vessel wall bulges out and creates a small pouch. Constant high-pressure blood flow to the pouch will cause the aneurysm to grow and potentially rupture.

Brain Stem Stroke

One of the more potentially devastating types of stroke occurs in the brain stem, which is responsible for involuntary functions of the body. A brain stem stroke is difficult to diagnose because patients don't experience typical stroke symptoms. Instead, they experience dizziness, loss of balance, and sudden vision changes, such as double vision. The brain stem controls the motor relays from the spine, balance, reflexes, coordination, breathing, heart rate, and blood pressure. A stroke in this region could impact someone's ability to breathe and regulate their heart rate. A brain stem stroke that damages the motor relays may lead to a condition called "locked-in syndrome." In this condition, the stroke survivor is fully alert and aware, but can move only their eyes. It is possible to recover from a brain stem stroke. In mild or moderate brain stem strokes, double vision and vertigo can resolve after a few weeks. Since the language centers are not affected, the stroke survivor has more success in participating actively in rehabilitation.

STROKE PREVENTION

Stroke is a preventable catastrophic condition and the leading cause of long-term adult disability. In the United States, someone has a stroke every 40 seconds. Every four minutes, someone dies of a stroke. Reducing the risk factors of stroke increases the chance of prevention. Stroke survivors have an increased risk of suffering from a second stroke.

There are both uncontrollable and controllable risk factors for stroke. Uncontrollable factors that increase your risk of stroke include age, sex, and race. People over the age of 55 are at higher risk. Men have a higher risk of stroke than women; however, women who suffer from a stroke when they are older have a higher risk of dying from a stroke than men. Also, African American people are 50 percent more likely to have a stroke than people of other ethnicities.

The American Heart Association recommends "Life's Simple 7" to reduce controllable risk factors for stroke:

1. **Manage blood pressure.** High blood pressure increases the strain on your heart, kidneys, and blood vessels.

2. **Stop smoking.** Lung damage from smoking decreases your body's ability to provide oxygen to the blood.

3. **Control cholesterol.** High cholesterol increases plaque buildup in your arteries, which can cause blood clots.

4. **Reduce blood sugar.** Controlling blood sugar reduces damage to your heart from the high concentration of glucose.

5. **Get active.** Daily exercise increases your stamina and improves the length and quality of life.

6. **Eat better.** A healthy diet reduces your risk for cardiovascular disease and stroke. A low-salt diet will improve blood pressure. Reducing your trans and saturated fat intake will help decrease cholesterol, and monitoring carbohydrate intake can reduce blood sugar.

7. **Lose weight if needed.** Unnecessary pounds increase the burden on the heart, lungs, and blood vessels.

In addition, treating the irregular heart rhythm called atrial fibrillation helps prevent the formation of blood clots that travel to the brain and cause a stroke. Active participation in managing controllable risk factors is the key to stroke prevention.

IS THIS A SIGN/SYMPTOM OF A STROKE?

An easy way to remember the signs or symptoms of a stroke is to use the acronym **BE FAST**. If you see these signs, even if they resolve on their own, call 911 right away.

"**BE**" stands for the symptoms of a posterior or brain stem stroke:

Balance: Sudden loss of balance, dizziness, or vertigo. Many things can cause dizziness and vertigo, but particularly when dizziness is coupled with the "E," it could mean a more serious condition, such as stroke.

Eyes: Sudden loss of vision in one or both eyes, or double vision. A gradual change in vision may not mean a stroke. Posterior strokes are difficult to diagnose because the symptoms can signal other medical conditions.

Though it can be one or the other, it is typically the combination of the loss of balance AND loss of vision that suggest a stroke.

Using the acronym **FAST** is an easy way to remember the most common signs of a stroke:

Face: Ask the person to smile or show you their teeth. Is their smile uneven? Does one side of their face droop downward?

Arm: Ask the person to lift both their arms. Are they able to keep both arms level or does one arm drift downward?

Speech: Ask the person to repeat a simple sentence. Does their speech sound slurred or strange? Are they having difficulty speaking?

Time: If the person is exhibiting any of these signs, even if they go away, call 911 right away. Tell the paramedics what time you first noticed these symptoms.

A stroke caused by an aneurysm rupture has a distinct set of symptoms. Symptoms of an aneurysm rupture include a sudden intense headache known as a "thunderclap headache." It is often described as "the worst headache ever." It can be accompanied by severe dizziness, inability to stand or walk, blurred or double vision, nausea or vomiting, or loss of consciousness.

Even after your loved one has a stroke, it is important to remember these signs and symptoms because stroke survivors are at a higher risk of suffering another stroke. Watch for the signs of a stroke so you can **BE FAST** and call 911.

DIAGNOSIS AND NEXT STEPS

When someone arrives in a hospital for a suspected stroke, things move very quickly. "Time is brain," after all, and increasing the chance for recovery is counted in minutes. Emergency room personnel will perform a variety of tasks in quick succession. Doctors will conduct a brief medical exam that focuses on neurologic changes. They will assess the patient's ability to move their arms and legs, speak, and track movement with their eyes. They'll also check the patient's coordination and their ability to feel sensation in different parts of their body. Meanwhile, nurses will draw blood, take vital signs, start intravenous lines (IVs), and assist with the neurological exam. They may also insert a urinary catheter or perform an electrocardiogram (ECG/EKG). As soon as possible, the patient is whisked away to radiology for a computerized tomography scan (CT scan) of the head. The CT scan will determine if the stroke is a hemorrhagic stroke, caused by bleeding in the brain, or an ischemic stroke, caused by a blood clot. The course of the patient's care is determined by these results.

If the CT scan shows a potential ischemic stroke, the goal of care is to restore blood flow to the brain as quickly as possible. Often, this means administering a potent clot-buster medication called "tissue plasminogen activator" (tPA). Not every patient is a candidate for tPA, though, especially those with a high risk for bleeding. Doctors must thoroughly review a patient's history and medication to determine if they could benefit from receiving intravenous tPA. Studies show that patients who receive tPA within four and a half hours of symptom onset have the best chance for recovery. The ability to receive tPA is why it is crucial to call 911 and come to the hospital as quickly as possible.

Ischemic stroke patients who have severe stroke symptoms may be suspected of having a blockage in one of the brain's major blood vessels. Doctors may order a CT angiogram (CTA) and a CT perfusion (CTP) scan of the brain. These results determine if someone is a candidate for a cerebral angiogram with thrombectomy. During a cerebral angiogram, the doctor inserts a long, thin, flexible tube called a catheter in a blood vessel in the patient's arm or leg. The catheter is threaded all the way to the person's brain, where dye is injected to map the blood vessels and determine where the blockage is. Once a clot is identified, the doctor uses a device inside the catheter to remove the clot. As the clot is removed, the vessel opens, restoring blood flow and oxygen. Studies have shown that people with blood clots in a major blood vessel of the brain can benefit from this procedure if it's performed within 24 hours of symptom onset.

For patients whose first CT scan of the head indicates a hemorrhagic stroke, treatment will follow a different path. Treatment for a hemorrhagic stroke focuses on quickly removing blood pooling in the brain and controlling the pressure building inside the skull. Depending on the location and size of the bleed, doctors may opt to drill a small hole in the skull to place a small tube to drain the blood and reduce pressure. For severe bleeds, a patient may be taken to surgery to open a wider hole in the skull and empty the pooling blood. Patients with aneurysms may undergo a surgical clipping or coiling to prevent the aneurysm from bleeding again. Surgeons may also remove or repair any malformations in the blood vessels to reduce future risk of rupture and stroke.

With either kind of stroke, after emergency treatment in the first 24 hours after the onset a stroke, your loved one may be admitted to the intensive care unit or a stroke unit for further monitoring. More tests may be ordered, such as magnetic resonance imaging (MRI) of the brain, echocardiogram, or carotid ultrasounds to determine potential causes of the stroke.

The next few days will be marked by visits from physical therapists, occupational therapists, and/or speech therapists to begin the road to recovery and rehabilitation. Dietitians and speech therapists may recommend specialized diets to accommodate any difficulty in swallowing. Most stroke patients will need rehabilitation following their hospital admission. More information on rehabilitation is found in chapter 3.

Case managers work with the patient and loved ones regarding discharge planning and arrangements for rehab facility placement, outpatient rehab services, or home health care. They will also arrange for delivery of durable medical equipment, such as walkers, wheelchairs, or shower chairs. Social workers will assist by providing community resources to support the patient and loved ones. Nurses will begin medication teaching for any new medications prescribed. Chaplains may also visit to offer spiritual support.

If you are in this situation, all this activity can often lead to strong emotions for you and your loved one, such as fear and confusion. Events are happening so quickly that it's easy for both you and your loved one to feel lost and confused. Your loved one may also experience frustration or anger at the sudden loss of their independence. The inability to function could trigger emotions such as helplessness and depression. The family of patients newly diagnosed with stroke may face fear for their loved ones during this period. Questions arise like *What will happen to them? Who will take care of them? How will we take care of them?* As roles shift and the caregiver role is taken on, a new caregiver may experience conflicted feelings, such as grief or loss of their former role. A sense of duty and responsibility can cause a caregiver to wrestle with this sudden shift in lifestyle.

Understand that your feelings and those of your loved one are entirely normal and natural. It is okay to be angry; it is okay to feel frustrated and lonely. You and your loved one must take the time to grieve and work through your emotions. Talk to each other and listen with an open heart and an open mind. This is a journey that you are facing together. Communicating honestly about your feelings is an essential foundation in this partnership. Learning how to work together, have fun together, and enjoy being part of each other's life is a journey under any circumstances, but never one that is taken alone.

WHAT TO ASK THE DOCTOR

- What caused the stroke? What kind of stroke is it?

- What kinds of tests will we need?

- What part of the brain did the stroke affect? What kind of changes can we expect? Are these changes likely to be permanent, or will they improve with time? With rehabilitation?

- What are my loved one's underlying medical conditions? Will they require other medical services?

- What can we do to promote recovery?

- Are there medications my loved one can take?

- What lifestyle changes can my loved one make?

- Are there any clinical trials my loved one can join?

HOW ARE YOU DOING?

I know that was a lot of information to process. I hope it helps you understand what may have happened in the hospital and why. Strokes are most often diagnosed in the hospital, and the speed at which things happened can leave you feeling breathless and lost. During the initial days following a stroke, your loved one may not remember details well, so it helps to understand what they went through and why. Remember, the reason things happened so fast is because time is brain. Knowing why this happened is a powerful tool for recovery and understanding.

The caregiver journey can be difficult. Some days will be better than others. You will experience days of doubt where you will question your ability to take care of your loved one or even if you're doing a good job. There will be days you celebrate, when your loved one can independently perform a task or communicate for the first time. My goal is to help walk you through those rough times. As they say, knowledge is power, and I will do my best to further your understanding so you won't feel so unsure of what to do.

Although you may feel that you should focus primarily on your loved one's needs, don't forget about yourself. Taking the time to address your needs can greatly help you on your journey. Carve out time every day—even 15 minutes—and spend it taking care of yourself. This will make you the best person and the best caregiver you can be.

Before you begin your caregiving journey, I have an assignment for you. Take a moment to ask yourself and reflect on the following questions/statements. Write your answers down on a sheet of paper or in a notebook.

- What scares me the most about the future?

- I am grateful for . . .

- What is the best thing my family did today?

- What is the best thing I did for myself today?

Now, close your eyes. Reach your arms up and stretch. Take a deep breath. You are not alone. You've got this.

One final note: If you don't have a notebook or journal, I encourage you to get one and keep a daily journal throughout your caregiving journey to help process your feelings.

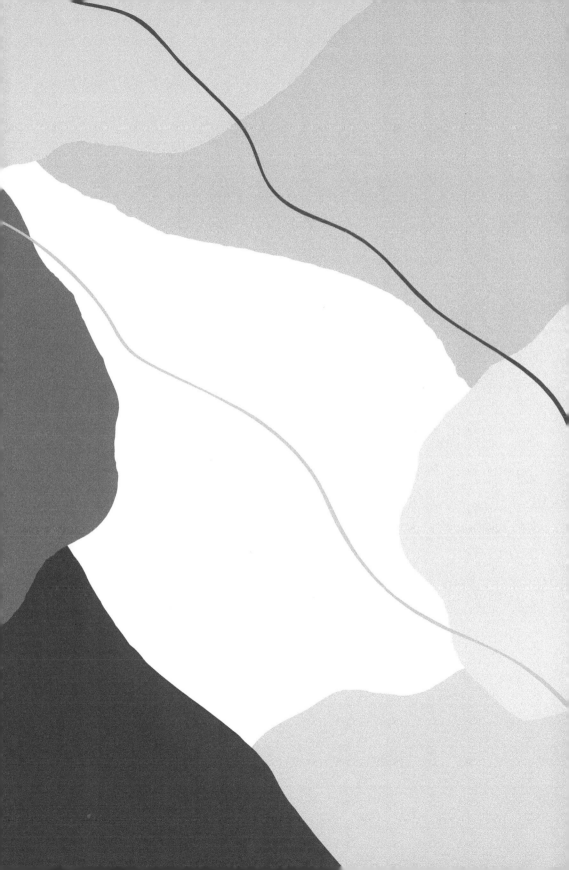

CHAPTER 2

A CAREGIVER'S JOURNEY BEGINS

Jerald

Jerald put a healthy dollop of shaving cream on his hand. He rubbed his hands together before slowly working the lather onto his father's cheeks and neck. The pale cream settled in the deep lines of his dad's craggy face.

He remembered as a young boy, watching his dad shave in the morning. He would watch how carefully his dad spread the shaving cream over his skin. His dad would grin at him in the mirror, then turn and playfully smear the leftover cream on Jerald's smooth cheeks.

"Mustache or goatee?" Dad would ask him. Jerald thought about it carefully. This was a serious question, after all.

"Mustache!" he declared.

His dad would proceed to shape the shaving cream on Jerald's little face to resemble a mustache. Dad meticulously curved the ends of his shaving cream mustache into a neat upward curve, creating a handlebar. Jerald laughed in delight. They took turns making faces at each other in the bathroom mirror.

Jerald looked at his dad in the mirror. It seemed like a long time since they had silly face contests in the mirror. His dad's skin was no longer young and smooth. Deep wrinkles framed his eyes and mouth. The left side of his mouth sagged and drooped since his stroke. Jerald turned to his dad and his lips quirked up in a lopsided grin. He picked up the razor.

"All right, Dad," he said. "Mustache or goatee?"

WHAT TO KEEP IN MIND

Allow time to adjust to your new roles. Both of you may have conflicting feelings. Taking time to process these feelings will foster understanding so you can be better together.

Involve your loved one in care decisions. Empower your loved one by encouraging them to be an active participant. Reassure them that their wishes are acknowledged and understood.

Communicate honestly. Develop understanding by sharing feelings and concerns together. Listen and recognize each other's needs, and, even more, be each other's advocate.

Promote independence. Encourage your loved one to do as much as they can do safely. They will appreciate the chance to regain some of their independence.

Create a plan together. Make a plan for activities they enjoy doing. Talk about what modifications may be needed. Don't be afraid to explore new activities they seem interested in.

Establish family support. Are there ways other family members can help? Can your brother take over Mom's care on Sundays so you can take a break? Can the grandkids visit Grandma to keep her company and make her smile? More people on the support team can make responsibilities easier to carry.

CHANGING RELATIONSHIPS

Caregiving is an act of service. To accept a caregiver's role begins a journey of taking care of your loved one's physical, emotional, spiritual, social, and financial needs. Becoming the caregiver of a loved one can often change the dynamic within a family unit. The stroke survivor and the caregiver experience a shift in roles and responsibilities.

The most common change in relationships is the reversal of roles. The stroke survivor moves from being the one taking care of the family to the one being taken care of. For example, a mother who traditionally was the caretaker of the family experiences a stroke and must now be taken care of by her adult children. This new way of life is a shared journey, and the stroke survivor and caregiver must lean on each other as "care partners."

The loss of independence can leave your loved one with feelings of frustration and helplessness as they struggle to adjust to their new role. Your loved one may have experienced physical changes that affect their ability to be independently mobile. The inability to use their dominant hand is incredibly frustrating. Your loved one may need assistance completing tasks that used to be easy. Tasks like peeling an orange, opening a jar, or even buttoning a shirt suddenly become daunting endeavors. Giving up autonomy and control can be difficult for your loved one. Some stroke survivors may feel that they are a burden on their family. Guilt can weigh heavily on their mind. Feelings of denial of their condition can lead to an unwillingness to accept help. As such, your loved one may overestimate their ability to do things for themself, which can be a potential safety hazard.

Caregivers also experience a significant shift in roles. In some cultures, the caregiver role is given to the women, with the expectation that they assume the majority of the responsibility. Up to 75 percent of all caregivers are women. On average, women will spend up to 50 percent more time providing care compared to a male caregiver.

Caregivers often have a heightened sense of responsibility and feel that they need to do "whatever needs to be done." This can include assisting with activities of daily living—feeding, dressing, bathing, toileting (using the toilet), and taking prescribed medications. Other tasks consist of household management, coordinating finances and medical care, and providing emotional support for their loved one. They may even feel a responsibility to be "the rock"—strong and dependable without fail. The added responsibility may feel overwhelming as a caregiver balances the care of their loved one with their own needs.

Family dynamics can have a significant influence on relationships between the stroke survivor and their caregivers. Sharing caregiver duties between family members has a dual benefit. When other members of the family get involved, this increases social interaction for your loved one and reduces feelings of loneliness and depression for everyone. By distributing care duties to other family members, you can ease the load and reduce the possibility of caregiver burnout.

Intimacy between spouses can also play a role in relationships. Stroke survivors may experience physical and emotional changes that decrease their desire for intimacy. Romantic relationships may also be strained for caregivers when they are stressed due to their new role and added responsibilities. It's important to remember that these feelings are normal, and recovery takes time. Physical intimacy and sex should be resumed only when both parties are ready. In the meantime, intimacy can come in many forms. There is more than one way to show that you love and care for each other.

As relationships evolve between stroke survivors and their caregivers, always try to remember that this is a journey taken together. You and your loved one are a team: partners in care. Communicating honestly and sharing decision-making will ensure a foundation of mutual trust and respect.

LONG-DISTANCE CAREGIVING

Most people think of caregiving as being by a loved one's side and tending to their needs. In some situations, a primary caregiver may not be able to live nearby. If you live more than an hour away from your loved one, you might be a long-distance caregiver. The responsibility of caring for your loved one from afar can present its own challenges.

Long-Distance Logistics

Not surprisingly, responding to your loved one's routine needs or emergency situations is more difficult across the miles. Your strategies for providing care will need to take into account how to provide as much independence as possible in the safest possible environment. Here are some top considerations:

Assess your loved one's care needs. What can they do independently? What do they need help with? How much help?

WHAT TO DO FIRST

Perform a home safety check. Check your loved one's home for safety hazards and implement safety measures to ensure that they can move around the house safely.

Make a list of what you need help with. Do you need help with finances, cleaning, and/or research? Who can help with transportation?

Create a local care team. Who are your loved one's local resources? Consider family, friends, neighbors, and their doctor or pharmacist. What local services can help, like cleaning companies, financial planners, or home care companies?

Establish a plan for regular communication. Set aside time to contact your loved one, via a visit, phone call, video call, text, or email. Network with family members to make a communication plan. When you are far away, regular contact helps to remind your loved one that you are thinking of them.

Use technology to your advantage. What devices can assist? Consider in-home monitoring and medical alert systems. What tools can be used to help your loved one around the house?

Post emergency contact lists in the home. Make an emergency contact list available in multiple locations, such as next to the phones, in bathrooms or bedrooms, or on the fridge. Update contact lists for friends and neighbors and your loved one's cell phone as contacts or numbers change.

Make an emergency kit. Assemble a bag of your loved one's clothes and toiletries that can be grabbed quickly in the event of an emergency. Include a list of their medications, emergency contact numbers, doctor contact numbers, and medical history. Station the bag in an easily accessible place so even emergency services or a neighbor can grab it if needed.

Conduct a thorough assessment of your loved one's home. Can they move safely around the house? Pay attention to changes in the flooring that could catch the tip of a walker or cane and pose a fall risk. Is the bathroom safe? Can they safely use stairs or steps? Are they able to contact help in an emergency?

Consider transportation. This includes doctor's appointments, pharmacies, or places that are important to your loved one, like social gatherings or religious services.

A long-distance caregiver's job revolves around two things: coordinating services and researching information. You'll need to research and arrange care for your loved one. Some suggestions:

- Seek out information about local resources, such as websites, community centers, or senior centers.

- Tap into your local Departments of Aging and Adult Services, Medical/Medicaid or Medicare office, Social Services office, or Veterans Affairs.

- Join local social media groups and find out about local services like meal or grocery delivery, housekeeping services, lawn care, or home repair services.

- Find out what agencies can provide care at home.

- Look into finding local doctors, specialists, or dentists. Where are the closest pharmacies and clinics? Where is the nearest emergency room or hospital?

- Consider which family members, friends, or neighbors you can rely on. If possible, include them in care planning for your loved one.

Use what you learn to build a network of services to support your loved one's independence.

Tending to Emotional Health from Afar

As a long-distance caregiver, it can be challenging to feel sufficiently connected. Of course, it's ideal to visit your loved one regularly. Visits allow you to connect on a deeper level and provide joy and comfort for your loved one. You can perform spot checks on their needs and home safety. Visits can be shared with other caregivers, friends, and family members. Also, asking others who live close by to visit expands your loved one's social circle. And a fresh set of eyes can pick up on things that you may have missed.

Visiting a loved one often may not be possible, so using other means to communicate can make it easier. This can be a quick phone call or text to check in. Video chat enables you to see each other, which allows for a better assessment of how your loved one is doing. Group video chats can include members of the family of all ages and from different locations. This connects your loved one with others and keeps other family members involved and in the loop. Email may be an option for stroke survivors who are able to type, and handwritten letters and greeting cards in the mail can be a lovely surprise for your loved one. By maintaining open lines of communication, in whatever form works best, you can stay aware of how your loved one is managing, while supporting their sense of independence.

It's understandable to be concerned about your loved one when you can't be there. Here are some gadgets that can be utilized to assist you and your loved one:

- In-home monitoring systems, such as cameras. These can monitor for safety, such as falls or even break-ins.

- For those who are uncomfortable having cameras in their home, some monitoring systems track sleep patterns, body temperature, or abnormal behavior.

- Medical alert systems or panic buttons. These can summon emergency help if needed.

- Smartwatches or fitness bands. These gadgets can track body functions, such as heart rate and calories burned.

- Automatic pill dispensers. These can assist your loved one in managing their medications.

- Smart home devices. Use them to regulate the temperature or turn on and off lights.

WORKING WITH A STROKE CARE TEAM

Have I mentioned that you are not alone? It takes a village to help a stroke survivor on the path to recovery. You and your loved one are the core team, and surrounding you are the healthcare professionals that make up the stroke care team. These team members provide professional advice and guidance for stroke recovery, and work together to support you and your loved one's needs.

As the caregiver, you are the advocate for your loved one, their voice when they cannot speak. Your communication with the care team is an important responsibility; in fact, caregivers are the best source of information regarding their loved one. Don't be afraid to speak up, and don't assume that your team members all have the same access to medical information. Just because something is "on file" or "in the chart" doesn't mean that clinics, hospitals, or doctors have complete medical information or documents.

It's also important to have a good relationship with your healthcare team. Not every team member will be a good fit for you or your loved one. If any team members aren't contributing to your loved one's recovery, you can try to work with them by discussing expectations and care goals. If problems can't be resolved, don't be afraid to switch out a team member for a different professional. It is always your choice who you want on the care team. Choose people who are right for you and your loved one; professionals you trust and feel like you can talk to. A stroke will impact your loved one for the rest of their life, and you need everyone on the team to have a shared vision.

You'll want to become familiar with each member of the healthcare team and the role they play. One team member may be better suited to support one aspect of recovery than another. Know your resources and who you can tap for help.

Primary Care Physician

The primary care physician (PCP) is responsible overall for managing your loved one's healthcare needs. They assess and monitor medical conditions and often recruit other team members to help, such as specialty physicians or rehabilitation therapists. The PCP often sees your loved one in a clinic, but some PCPs have privileges to manage care for their patients while in a hospital. It helps maintain continuity of care when a PCP can cover both clinic and hospital visits. Some clinics and hospitals also incorporate telehealth services to assist PCPs in following up on their patients.

Neurologist

Neurologists are specialty doctors trained in managing medical conditions of the brain and nervous system. Some neurologists specialize in specific conditions, such as stroke, dementia, Alzheimer's, or epilepsy. Neurologists are an excellent resource for answering questions on the care and treatment of stroke.

Neurosurgeon

Neurosurgeons are specially trained in surgical procedures of the brain and spine. If your loved one underwent a surgical procedure such as an aneurysm repair, they may follow up with the neurosurgeon, who will manage care concerning their surgery.

Nurses

Nurses are the heart and hands of health care. They are your greatest champion and source for help. You will find nurses in the hospital, at the acute rehabilitation facility, and in clinics. Nurses can educate you and your loved one on many subjects, including your loved one's medical condition and medication management. Don't hesitate to ask your nurse for help. They can often provide information or help get you what you need.

Case Manager

A case manager is a nurse who evaluates your loved one and collaborates with you to develop a healthcare plan. In the hospital, case managers focus on carrying out a safe discharge plan. They arrange for home care or placement in acute rehabilitation facilities or skilled nursing facilities. Case managers set up delivery of equipment such as wheelchairs or home oxygen. When you are home, your insurance company's case manager is in charge of phone call follow-ups and answering your questions regarding insurance coverage and options.

Social Workers

Clinical social workers are trained in assessing, diagnosing, treating, and preventing emotional and behavioral disturbances and mental illness. Social workers are trained in psychotherapy and connect people with their community. A clinical social worker can help you obtain community resources and support services for your loved one. Like case managers, clinical social workers assist both in the hospital and through your insurance carrier.

Physical Therapist

The physical therapist is a member of the rehabilitation team. They focus on the rehabilitation of gross motor skills, such as functional mobility and body positioning. Physical therapists help your loved one improve movement and manage pain. They train caregivers on the safe handling of a loved one and exercises to do with the loved one to regain mobility and functional independence.

Occupational Therapist

The occupational therapist focuses on the rehabilitation of fine motor movement. They specialize in treating things that prevent people from performing activities of daily living (ADLs) or working. For example, an occupational therapist may work with your loved one on dressing, feeding, or brushing their teeth. Therapy may also include skills to support returning to work, such as grasping, typing, lifting small objects, and other fine motor movements.

Speech Therapist

Speech-language pathologists, or speech therapists, treat communication, cognitive (thinking, reasoning, or remembering), and swallowing disorders. They work with your loved one on regaining the ability to speak or to safely swallow their food. Speech therapists may recommend modified diets if a stroke survivor has dysphagia (difficulty swallowing food). If your loved one's stroke affected their memory or cognition, a speech therapist can help.

Dietitian

Dietitians work closely with speech therapists to accommodate diets in response to difficulty swallowing. A dietitian will ensure that your loved one is receiving the proper nutrition to meet their needs. In cases where a stroke survivor completely loses the ability to swallow, a dietitian may recommend a feeding tube. A dietitian is also a terrific resource to ask questions about nutrition and supplements.

Chaplain

If you or your loved one seeks spiritual counsel in the hospital, don't hesitate to request a visit from the hospital chaplain. While most of the healthcare team focuses on physical recovery, maintaining a strong spiritual connection can be very powerful. At home, you can feed your souls by connecting with your local church, synogague, mosque, or spiritual advisor. Fellow members of your faith community can provide emotional and spiritual support for both you and your loved one.

HOW ARE YOU DOING?

As a new caregiver, you've got many emotions to unpack. This may have been something that you were expecting, or perhaps it's something that came on very suddenly. Mixed feelings are expected, as grief over the loss of your former lifestyle clashes with your sense of duty to your loved one.

The caregiver role can be overwhelming. As a new caregiver, please take the time to process these emotions. If you don't come to terms with your feelings, you won't be able to function. You're not alone, however, because your loved one is grappling with similar conflicting emotions. They may be experiencing feelings of hopelessness, frustration, or guilt about being a burden.

To successfully function as care partners, communicate with each other honestly about your feelings, fears, and frustrations. Take as much time as you need. When you are ready, talk about how the two of you can support each other emotionally. Let your loved one help you, too.

If your loved one has difficulty speaking due to their stroke, a communication board can be a lifesaver. A communication board has pictures, words, and letters that your loved one can point to and express their thoughts, feelings, and needs. You can purchase them online or create your own to fit your loved one's situation. They are also available as apps for your phone or tablet.

Now I have one assignment just for you. Give yourself permission to cry. You don't have to be strong all the time, and you don't have to hold it in. Sometimes a good cry can help you let go of those emotions.

HOW TO WORK WITH YOUR CARE TEAM

Be honest, open, and patient. Keep communication lines open with the healthcare team, and don't be afraid to advocate for your loved one or express how you feel. Getting support will be easier if people understand the situation.

Use "I" statements instead of "you" statements. If conflict arises with a team member, saying "I feel angry" instead of "You make me angry" communicates your feelings without blaming others and making them defensive.

Clarify what you hear. When you talk to your care team, repeat what you hear and make sure you understand instructions and information.

Write it down. Writing down questions before speaking with your healthcare team will keep you more organized and prevent you from forgetting something important. Taking notes during meetings is also helpful.

Show your appreciation. Thank friends, family, or members of the healthcare team for their help. Gratitude can go a long way in making others feel good about being on your team.

WHAT TO ASK YOUR CARE TEAM

- What kind of specialists will we need?

- What is your treatment philosophy?

- What equipment can we use to make things easier?

- How can we reduce the risk of another stroke?

- Do you have any resources that may help us?

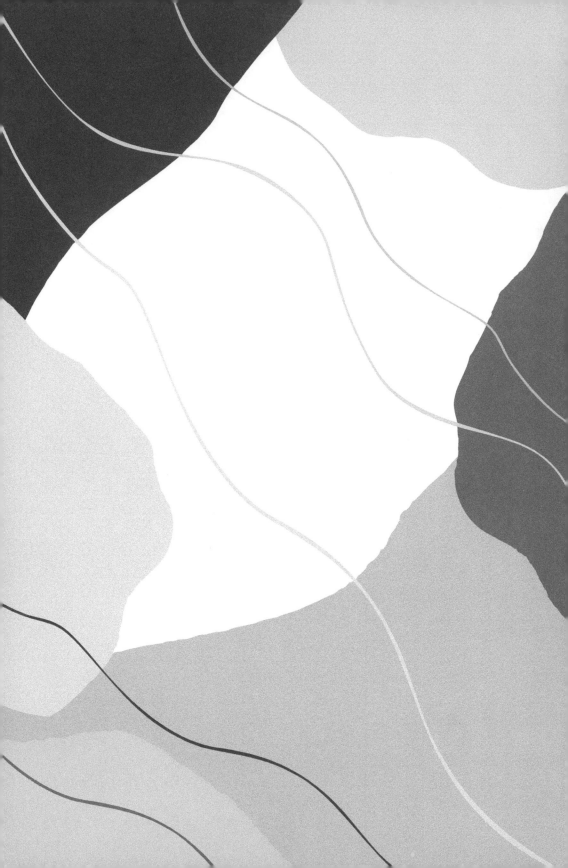

PART TWO

CARING FOR SOMEONE RECOVERING FROM A STROKE

CHAPTER 3

STROKE RECOVERY AND REHABILITATION

Amina

A mina looked at herself in the mirror. She could see the left side of her face perfectly, but the right side of her face was one big black spot. Amina had a type of visual impairment that allowed her to see everyone else's face completely, but only half of her own. On top of that, Amina had tunnel vision. The top, bottom, and sides of her visual field were black. She moved through the world as if she were always looking through a telescope.

Amina had a stroke last year, just a few months after her 32nd birthday. Most people wouldn't know that she had a stroke, because there were no obvious signs to others; however, it damaged her memory and her visual processing center. She didn't have any motor deficits and could use her arms and legs without any problems. But Amina suffered from short-term memory loss. She had to make sure she wrote everything down. In the weeks following her stroke, she would forget conversations after 15 minutes. These were things no one else could see. To the world, Amina was a normal 33-year-old woman.

Thankfully, her rehabilitation therapy sessions were helping. Amina had been seeing a speech therapist three times a week to work on improving her memory and vision. Now she could keep track of conversation topics and recall people she met months ago. If she closed her eyes tight and then opened them quickly, for a split second, she could see everything before it narrowed to tunnel vision.

Amina sighed as she looked at her face in the mirror. Things were getting better, but she still had a long road ahead of her. Therapy was hard, and she was trying her best to stay motivated. She looked at the black spot that was supposed to be the right side of her face. "I really miss doing my makeup." She glanced at her makeup bag sitting on the bathroom counter. "One day, I will," she promised herself.

THE RECOVERY JOURNEY

For healthcare professionals, recovery from stroke is about the long game. It's not "I need to cure your illness" or "I need to save your life," but instead "I need to preserve your quality of life in the future and prevent another stroke." The backbone of stroke care is rehabilitation therapy. Stroke survivors can experience multiple combinations of deficits and must receive therapy to regain what they have lost.

The rehabilitation road is a long one, and the timeline for recovery varies. It is vital to start rehabilitation immediately after the stroke. Rehabilitation therapy is critical for all stroke survivors, but it is different for everyone. Some survivors can recover most of their function, but others with severe strokes may have limited recovery. Rehabilitation does not reverse the damage caused by a stroke but instead creates new pathways in the brain (neuroplasticity) and helps a stroke survivor restore the best health and function possible.

Rehabilitation goals include:

- Improving function

- Promoting independence

- Managing deficits

- Reducing disability

- Building strength and endurance

- Learning strategies to compensate for deficits

- Returning to work if possible

Stroke rehabilitation begins in the hospital, immediately following a diagnosis of stroke. Those who start rehabilitation therapy early have shown a greater chance of recovery. Studies have also shown that the best chance of recovery occurs within the first year following a stroke. Rehabilitation therapy involves a lot of repetition and practice. Stroke survivors are relearning how to do things or retraining cognitive functions. It's important to know that a plateau in progress is normal, and not necessarily a sign of stopping. Recovery and healing can still be possible in the years following a stroke.

A typical rehabilitation team will consist of a doctor, nurse, physical therapist, occupational therapist, and speech therapist. Depending on the needs, the team may also include a case manager, social worker, or dietitian. The rehabilitation team evaluates your loved one and implements a plan of care. Goals are set, and progress is measured by how well a stroke survivor meets specific goals (for example, walk 30 feet with a walker with minimal assistance). Based on the progress, therapists will make recommendations for home equipment. Recommendations can include facilities or services for continuing rehabilitation.

Family and caregiver training is another large part of rehabilitation therapy. This training includes safe handling of your loved one at home, such as helping your loved one move safely from bed to chair. Therapists will show you how to perform these tasks to minimize strain on your body and avoid hurting yourself. You may also learn how to help your loved one with home exercises.

Successful overall rehabilitation depends on:

- Location and extent of damage caused by the stroke

- The rehabilitation team's proficiency

- Cooperation and support by caregivers, family, and friends

- Motivation of the stroke survivor during rehabilitation

- Commitment to the therapy program and dedication to continuing rehabilitation at home

COMMON REHABILITATION THERAPIES

Rehabilitation therapy plays a large role in stroke recovery. Without rehabilitation therapy, your loved one will not regain lost function. But therapy isn't just about regaining lost function. It is also to build

WHAT TO SAY TO YOUR LOVED ONE

"You are a stroke survivor." Using the term "stroke victim" often has negative connotations. Using "stroke survivor" or even "stroke warrior" is much more encouraging—surely that is who they are!

"Take your time." After a stroke, your loved one is relearning things. Be patient—they may feel like they are learning something for the first time.

"Let's take a break." It's essential to stimulate the brain to promote healing, but too much stimulation can drain energy. Reduce background noise and unnecessary distractions as much as you can.

WHAT TO DO AS A CAREGIVER

Encourage daily exercise. By working rehabilitation exercises into your loved one's day, those exercises will encourage the brain to rewire itself while building and maintaining strength and endurance.

Stick to the plan. A solid commitment to the rehabilitation program will enhance recovery. Make a deal with your loved one to stick to the plan together.

Be just helpful enough. Stroke survivors need to do as much as they can on their own. If they are struggling, only help if they ask or if you see it's necessary. Foster as much independence as you can.

Celebrate the small stuff. Small milestones are just as important as big ones; celebrate them all. Any progress is a step in the right direction.

Stay the course. Times will get tough, and progress may seem slow. Keep pushing. The brain is capable of recovery for years after a stroke.

WHAT TO ASK THE DOCTOR

- What can we expect during recovery?
- What type of rehab is needed and for how long?
- Where is the best place to continue recovery?

strength and coordination and to keep the body from deteriorating and growing weak. Your loved one's deficits will determine which therapists will be assigned.

There are three major types of rehabilitation therapy: physical therapy, occupational therapy, and speech therapy. Each discipline focuses on care and treatment of specific deficits. Stroke survivors benefit the most when receiving multiple therapy types.

Caregivers are an integral part of recovery. Expect to be an active participant during your loved one's therapy. It's important for you to learn these techniques as well, to support rehabilitation and recovery at home. Don't be afraid to jump in and learn what you can from the therapists.

Physical Therapy

Physical therapy targets functional mobility. A physical therapist will address deficits such as paralysis, diminished motor control and coordination, and sensory disturbances. Physical therapy goals support the recovery of general mobility.

Your loved one may learn about bed mobility, such as how to move around and position in bed. These exercises can include rolling side to side or repositioning from supine (lying flat on back) to a sitting position. Using splints or orthotics can support proper positioning. Your loved one may practice how to maintain their balance while sitting, standing, and reaching.

Other exercises focus on the ability to transfer from bed to chair and back again. Your loved one may learn how to sit and stand safely. As a caregiver, a physical therapist may instruct you on how to safely use transfer devices like slider boards and lifts to assist your loved one at home.

Physical therapy may also focus on walking or wheelchair mobility. Your loved one may learn how to propel themself in a wheelchair. For stroke survivors with more mobility in their legs, a physical therapist will initiate gait training. Gait training focuses on strengthening the legs and relearning how to walk, using assistive devices such as walkers or canes, and navigating stairs and ramps.

Another goal of physical therapy is to prevent muscle loss and weakness. Exercises will focus on building strength and maintaining flexibility. Stroke survivors suffering from paralysis of their limbs can develop a permanent form of stiffness called "contractures." Joints become "frozen" and immobile and cannot bend without causing discomfort or pain. Stroke survivors who are bedridden are especially prone to developing contractures. More information about paralysis and contractures is in chapter 5.

Occupational Therapy

Occupational therapists focus on retraining mobility related to activities of daily living (ADLs). These therapy exercises are geared toward feeding, grooming, bathing, dressing, toileting, and sexual functioning.

Stroke survivors who have lost function in one of their arms will learn hemi-technique. Your loved one will learn how to complete tasks one-handed. Have you ever tried to put on a long-sleeved shirt one-handed? Give it a try. After you've struggled to put on the shirt, ask the occupational therapist to show you how to do it and how best to help your loved one.

An occupational therapist may introduce your loved one to assistive devices that can help them perform ADLs. Some devices include sock aids, long-handled shoehorns, and button hooks. Shower chairs, bath boards, and handheld shower heads can make bathing easier. Bowls with suction-cup bottoms and utensils with large, easy-to-grip handles can promote independence while eating.

Speech Therapy

Speech therapy concentrates on the treatment of swallowing disorders, cognitive impairments, and speech and language deficits. Speech therapists can treat cognitive deficits, such as memory loss and visual perception issues, like those chronicled in Amina's story at the beginning of the chapter.

When a stroke survivor has difficulty swallowing (dysphagia), a speech therapist aims to decrease choking risk. Dysphagia therapy includes exercises that strengthen and coordinate swallowing muscles in the throat. Techniques such as where to place food inside the mouth or how to position the head and body to help with swallowing may be taught A speech therapist may recommend changes in food consistencies to aid in swallowing. See chapter 6 for more information about dysphagia.

Speech therapists treat speech and language deficits (aphasia) in order to help improve communication. Your loved one may work on exercises to improve their articulation and breath support (how to move air to form words). Therapy for language deficits begins with simple activities that grow in complexity over time. More information about aphasia can be found in chapter 5.

For cognitive deficits, a speech therapist will employ strategies to improve short- and long-term memory, attention, information processing, problem-solving, and organization. Cognitive exercises address deficits we can't see. Activities can include context-related problem-solving, reasoning, or organization of tasks of increasing complexity. Training may target executive functions, such as goal-setting, initiating plans or actions, self-awareness, inhibition (stopping yourself from performing an action), and self-monitoring and evaluation.

WHERE TO REHAB

After a stroke, rehabilitation often begins in the hospital. The social worker or case manager will work with you to determine the best place for continued recovery after discharge. Some stroke survivors may return home, but others may benefit from rehabilitation facilities. Your loved one's ability to engage in therapy will play a critical role in their rehabilitation plan. The American Stroke Association (ASA) recommends participation in rehabilitation for as long as possible.

Stroke survivors with multiple deficits who can actively participate in therapy may benefit from staying at an inpatient rehabilitation facility for a few weeks and engaging in a structured rehabilitation program. Here they will participate in at least three hours of therapy per day, up to five or six days a week. Treatment can be any combination of physical, occupational, and speech therapy sessions. Often, sessions are a

WHAT TO SAY TO YOUR LOVED ONE

"We're a team." Reassure your loved one that you are care partners. Your support will reduce their anxiety and frustration.

"That looked hard. You did great!" As a caregiver, you are their number-one cheerleader. A little encouragement can go a long way to motivate your loved one.

"Let's get some ice cream." When your loved one is feeling unmotivated, give them an incentive. Offer a small treat or activity as a reward.

HOW TO SUPPORT REHABILITATION

Make a game out of it. Incorporate fun in rehabilitation activities. An internet search for "stroke rehab games" can pull up games that promote stroke recovery.

Keep the mind sharp. Brain teasers, such as puzzles, card games, and crosswords, will enhance problem-solving and memory skills. Exercising cognitive skills is just as important as focusing on physical recovery.

Get creative. Promote recovery through creative activities, such as painting, doing arts and crafts, or listening to music.

Encourage mindfulness. Relaxation, meditation, and mindfulness are easily accessible through apps or internet videos. Reducing stress and anxiety is a great way to recharge; plus, it's an activity you can do together.

WHAT TO ASK THE THERAPIST

- What exercises can we do at home?

- Can we have a set of written instructions on how to perform the exercises?

- May I make an audio or video recording of you explaining or demonstrating these exercises?

- What apps or games can we use to help recovery?

mix of individual therapy and group therapy. Inpatient rehabilitation facilities generally include 24-hour doctor supervision and nursing care.

Skilled nursing facilities (SNFs) are appropriate for stroke survivors who need some nursing care and a less intensive rehabilitation program. An SNF may be an option if your loved one can't tolerate three or more hours of therapy per day. Rehabilitation services offered at an SNF require fewer hours of participation.

Long-term acute care (LTAC) facilities are for stroke survivors who require 24-hour nursing support. An LTAC may be recommended if your loved one is too ill to participate in aggressive rehabilitation therapy and may benefit from a limited therapy program.

Once a stroke survivor goes home, rehabilitation services will depend on their functional abilities. Therapy may include outpatient visits to rehabilitation therapy two or three times per week. Your loved one would need transportation to and from their appointments. Feeding, cognitive issues, residual weakness, high-balance activities, strengthening and conditioning, and gross and fine motor rehabilitation can all be addressed with outpatient rehabilitation therapy.

For stroke survivors who only need treatment from a single rehabilitation specialist, home health services may be an option. Home health care can also be helpful if transportation is not readily available or your loved one has serious mobility issues. Home health services are often dependent on insurance coverage, and your loved one will need to meet certain criteria to qualify. Home health care can address simple mobility issues but is not recommended for more aggressive therapy. Access to specialized equipment is not possible for rehabilitation therapy at home; however, your loved one will learn strategies for working within their own environment. The therapist can make recommendations during a home safety evaluation for home modifications and care.

WHAT TO SAY TO YOUR LOVED ONE

"What do you think?" This important question engages your loved one in the decision-making process. Decisions about their care should be made together whenever possible.

"Can you repeat that?" Stroke survivors may need time to process a situation. Ask them to repeat what they understand to make sure everyone is on the same page.

"Let's make a visitation/communication plan." If your loved one is in a facility, create a visitation or communication plan together so they can feel supported while away from home.

HOW TO GET GOOD REHAB

Find out what type of rehabilitation care insurance will cover. The case manager in a hospital, rehabilitation facility, or insurance provider can assist with this.

Do your research. Search for an accredited rehabilitation facility. The Commission on the Accreditation of Rehabilitation Facilities (CARF) is an international accrediting body. Visit their website for a list of facilities near you. Ask the case manager for their recommendations and read online reviews.

Scout the site. Visit prospective rehabilitation facility sites. Don't be afraid to ask staff questions about their facility and the care that's provided.

Continue being their advocate. Nobody cares for your loved one like you. Stay aware of how things are going for your loved one at the facility and make sure they are getting what they need.

Chronicle the journey. Take pictures, videos, or notes of your loved one's rehabilitation progress and celebrate their successes with the family. Seeing and acknowledging how far they have come can be a great source of encouragement for everyone.

WHAT TO ASK THE THERAPIST

- How much can my loved one participate in rehab services?

- Is this facility certified to take care of people with stroke-related issues?

- How much rehab therapy will my loved one receive, and in which areas? How intensive will it be?

- How do you measure progress?

- How do we prevent falls?

- Do you have any tips and tricks?

- How can we prepare our home?

HOW ARE YOU DOING?

Setting the stage for your loved one's rehabilitation journey is one of the first steps. What to do next and deciding how to form a therapy plan can be scary. You may be intimidated thinking about what the future will bring. Take a breath, and lean on your healthcare team's professional advice. Don't be afraid to ask questions. They will have helpful knowledge and recommendations on the services your loved one will need.

There are many decisions you and your loved one will make together on this journey, and no one starts out as an expert. The important thing is to learn and grow together from your mistakes. Even if you make a mistake, your loved one will still love and support you.

The start of any rehabilitation is often difficult for your loved one, too. Relearning new skills is a daily challenge. These new skills may seem easy to other people, but for them, it can be an overwhelming task. Your loved one may need encouragement and emotional support. Being the constant cheerleader, however, can place a mental strain on a caregiver as well. Sometimes, mental exhaustion can be more draining than physical.

Maintaining your mental health is an essential factor, and you'll want to manage your stress. If you're feeling overwhelmed, don't be afraid to take a minute for yourself. It's okay to walk away for a few minutes to collect your thoughts and emotions. If you can't take care of yourself, you're no good to your loved one.

Take some time to practice mindfulness. Search YouTube for "guided meditation." Take a few minutes and try videos on guided meditation or breathing exercises. Some free apps are available on a smartphone or tablet that you can try as well. A mindfulness practice can become a valuable ritual to help you collect your thoughts and relax your mind. Managing stress and making time for your own self-care will make you a better caregiver.

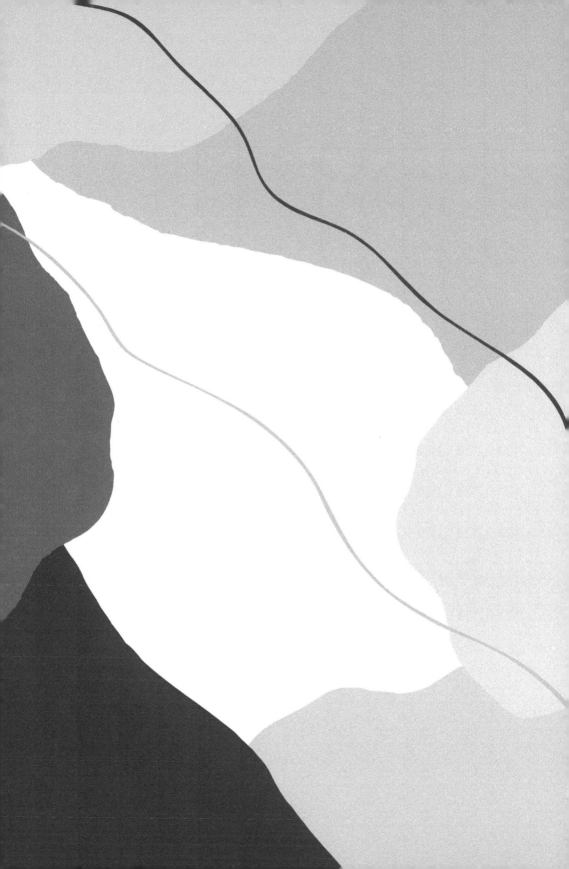

CHAPTER 4

MEDICATIONS AND TREATMENTS

Jade

Jade carefully opened the pill organizer lid marked "Tuesday Morning." She shook out the pills inside and counted: one, two, three, four. Satisfied, she placed them in the pill crusher and twisted the lid back and forth. The pills cracked and popped until they became a fine multicolored powder. She tapped the powder into a small cup and set it down on a tray. She placed a cup of applesauce, a pudding cup, and a spoon next to the crushed medication. Then she picked up the tray and walked into the living room where her dad was watching TV.

"I've got your meds," she announced.

Her dad made a face. Well, technically, he made half a face. Half of his face drooped down while the other half wrinkled in displeasure.

"It tastes nasty mixed in applesauce," he complained.

"I brought you chocolate pudding, too. It's sugar-free," Jade reassured him. Dad's stroke left him with difficulty swallowing. All his medications needed to be crushed and mixed in something thick enough for him to swallow without choking.

"Can't I have it in ice cream?" Dad tried to bargain. "They have sugar-free ice cream. I can have that."

Jade considered it. "Okay, I'll pick some up when I go to the store. We can try it in ice cream next time." She picked up the applesauce cup in one hand and the chocolate pudding in the other. She shook them enticingly. "Applesauce or pudding?"

"Pudding," Dad grunted in disgust.

Jade opened the pudding cup and dumped the crushed medication inside. Gently, she stirred it with a spoon. "Okay, now open wide," she teased.

"It better be chocolate ice cream next time," Dad grumbled and opened his mouth.

COMMON MEDICATIONS AND TREATMENTS

Your loved one may be prescribed certain medications to help with stroke recovery or prevent a recurrent stroke. Medication treatment depends on the type of stroke. In this section are basic descriptions of the most common medications that may be prescribed for both ischemic and hemorrhagic stroke. Other drugs may be available, and this list is not all-inclusive.

Please consult your doctor before starting any medications or supplements. Some vitamins, supplements, and herbal remedies may affect prescribed medications. Let your doctor know which medications or supplements your loved one may be taking. Be sure only to give the prescribed dose of medications, and don't stop medications unless advised by your doctor.

When reading a medication label, know that generic names are usually listed first. Some medications have brand names, but your insurance may only cover the generic brand. Don't worry; generic medications have the same effectiveness as their equivalent brand. The doctor or pharmacist can tell you about any differences between generic and brand-name medications.

Antiplatelets

Antiplatelet medications are blood thinners that prevent platelets from sticking together. This will prevent clots from forming and growing. Antiplatelets are often given to ischemic stroke patients to stop a blood clot from forming that could cause a second stroke.

The most commonly prescribed antiplatelet is aspirin, or acetylsalicylic acid. If your loved one is prescribed aspirin, it should be taken with food since it can bother the stomach. Other antiplatelet drugs include clopidogrel (Plavix), prasugrel (Effient), and ticagrelor (Brilinta). In some instances, your loved one may be prescribed two antiplatelet medications.

Note: Someone taking an antiplatelet medication will take a little longer to stop bleeding if they get scratched or cut. Bumps turn into bruises quickly and small skin tears can ooze. People with diabetes who check their blood sugar with finger sticks will bleed a little longer. Be sure to hold pressure on any bleeding a little longer than usual.

When taking over-the-counter medication for pain, acetaminophen (Tylenol) is preferable to ibuprofen (Motrin or Advil). Ibuprofen has some mild blood-thinning properties that could increase the risk for bleeding for those on blood thinner medication.

Anticoagulants

Anticoagulants are a more powerful blood thinner than antiplatelets. They work on the clotting factors in the blood to prevent clot formation. Anticoagulants are often prescribed to stroke survivors with atrial fibrillation who are at risk for blood clots. Anticoagulants prevent new blood clots from forming and keep existing blood clots from getting larger. Common anticoagulants are warfarin (Coumadin), apixaban (Eliquis), dabigatran (Pradaxa), or rivaroxaban (Xarelto). If they take an anticoagulant, your loved one may need to get routine blood tests to make sure their blood isn't too thin or too thick.

Note: The risk for bleeding is higher in someone who is taking an anticoagulant. Simple fixes can help with this. Using a soft-bristled toothbrush can reduce gum bleeding. An electric shaver can reduce nicks and cuts. Avoid eating dark leafy vegetables, such as kale, collard greens, broccoli, or spinach. Vitamin K found in dark leafy vegetables may counteract the effects of the anticoagulant. Consult your doctor or dietitian about what foods to avoid while taking an anticoagulant.

Both antiplatelets and anticoagulants carry a risk of bleeding. Gastrointestinal (GI) bleeding may occur, so call the doctor or go to the emergency room if you notice any of the following:

- blood in the stools or urine

- stools that look like black tar

- blood in vomit

- vomit that looks like coffee grounds

Statins

You may be familiar with "good" cholesterol and "bad" cholesterol. Good cholesterol, or high-density lipoprotein (HDL) cholesterol, transports cholesterol to the liver for removal from your body. Bad, low-density lipoprotein (LDL) cholesterol takes cholesterol to the blood vessels, where it can build up and form plaque.

Statins are medications that reduce LDL cholesterol. These drugs block an enzyme that your body uses to make cholesterol and plaque. Plaque can clog blood vessels and increase the chance of strokes.

Some common statins are atorvastatin (Lipitor), rosuvastatin (Crestor), and simvastatin (Zocor). Statins are typically taken once a day. Most statins are more effective when taken at night when your body creates the most cholesterol, but some extended-release statins can be taken at any time of day.

Note: Avoid grapefruit juice while taking statins. Grapefruit juice can cause the statin to remain in your body longer, causing a drug buildup. This increases the risk of liver damage, muscle breakdown, or kidney failure. Common side effects of statins include muscle aches, nausea, and headache.

Antihypertensives

The management of hypertension (high blood pressure) plays a significant role in stroke prevention. High blood pressure can contribute to clot formation due to chunks of plaque breaking off the inside of your blood vessels. Chronic high blood pressure can weaken the walls of blood vessels and form aneurysms. It can also cause ruptures in the blood vessels, leading to a hemorrhagic stroke. An estimated 51 percent of stroke deaths around the world are attributed to high blood pressure.

A diuretic, sometimes known as a "water pill," reduces blood pressure by helping the kidneys eliminate excess salt and water and reducing overall blood volume. Common diuretics include chlorothiazide (Diuril) or hydrochlorothiazide (Hydrodiuril), spironolactone (Aldactone), and furosemide (Lasix).

Note: Diuretics make you urinate, so avoid taking them at night or before bedtime. Stroke survivors with bladder control problems may require more frequent trips to the bathroom or adult diapers. Since you may lose potassium in the urine, eating foods high in potassium, like bananas or sweet potatoes, can help prevent leg cramps, muscle weakness, and fatigue.

Four common blood pressure medication types are angiotensin-converting enzyme (ACE) inhibitors, angiotensin II receptor blockers (ARBs), beta blockers, and calcium channel blockers. These drug types work on different parts of the blood vessels and heart to reduce blood pressure.

ACE inhibitors and ARBs lower blood pressure by helping expand blood vessels to let more blood through and thereby lower blood pressure. ACE inhibitors have names that end in "-pril," such as benazepril (Lotensin), enalapril (Vasotec), and lisinopril (Prinivil, Zestril). ARBs have names that end in "-sartan" like losartan (Cozaar) and valsartan (Diovan).

Note: ACE inhibitors can cause some people to have a dry, persistent cough, in which case a doctor may prescribe an ARB instead.

Beta blockers are drugs that block the chemicals that stimulate your heart, causing the heart to beat more slowly and with less force. The blood pressure goes down because blood is circulating more slowly. Beta-blocker medication names end in "-lol," such as atenolol (Tenormin), metoprolol (Lopressor), and propranolol (Inderal).

Note: Due to the lowered heart rate, your loved one may feel dizzy or lightheaded. Let the doctor know if this occurs so you can discuss the possible risks and benefits of changing the dosage or discontinuing the beta blocker, if necessary.

Calcium channel blockers lower blood pressure by blocking the exchange of calcium. With less calcium being exchanged to drive muscle contraction, the heart beats with less force and the blood vessels relax, reducing blood pressure. Some calcium channel blockers have names that end in "-pine," like amlodipine (Norvasc), and nifed-ipine (Adalat). Other calcium channel blockers, such as diltiazem (Cardizem) or verapamil (Calan SR), may also be prescribed.

Note: As with statins, grapefruit juice should be avoided with certain calcium channel blockers. Grapefruit juice can interact with certain calcium channel blockers and affect blood pressure and heart rate, causing dizziness and headaches.

MEDICATION SUPPORT

Stroke survivors may face challenges with medication management. Trouble swallowing or cognitive issues can make it difficult for them to take their meds. Medications can also be expensive, since insurance coverage for prescriptions varies. For a stroke survivor living alone, transportation and physical limitations can make it challenging to get medications filled.

With regard to swallowing, crushing pills and mixing them with food can make the medication easier to swallow. Applesauce is the most common food to mix medications in, but experiment with other similar textures such as pudding, yogurt, sherbet, or ice cream. Allow time for your loved one to swallow; they may need to swallow several times before it will go down.

With regard to cost, don't be afraid to comparison shop or check online pharmacies. Generic brands are often less expensive than brand-name medications. Some drug companies offer patient assistance programs that provide discounts on select drugs. If the prescription is expensive, ask the pharmacy if there are coupons, and/or contact the doctor for advice and ask if there are cheaper alternatives.

Limited mobility or transportation can also make it difficult for your loved one to get their prescriptions refilled. Some local pharmacies and mail-order pharmacies take phone and online orders and offer delivery. If mobility or transportation are an issue, consider having medications delivered to the home, or have someone pick up the prescriptions for your loved one.

WHAT TO SAY ABOUT MEDICATION

"Time to take your medication." Sometimes stroke survivors have a hard time remembering when to take their pills. Incorporating a medication schedule into the daily routine can help keep your loved one on track.

"How do you feel when you take that drug?" Some drugs will have side effects, and your loved one may not mention how they feel. Prompt them to examine how the drug makes them feel to identify any potential issues.

"Are you ready for the next one?" Your loved one may need extra time to swallow medicine, so allow time between each one.

"I understand that you don't want to take your medication. Help me understand why." Sometimes people don't want to take medication. Listen and validate their feelings. They may be refusing their medications because of side effects, lack of knowledge, or another reason that may shed light on things.

"How would you like to take your medicine?" Encourage active participation in your loved one's medication treatment by asking their preferences. Do they prefer to take their medication with their meal or after the meal? Crushed in applesauce or yogurt? In one spoonful or multiple?

WHAT TO DO ABOUT MEDICATION

Find a primary care doctor you can trust. A good primary care doctor can coordinate with all the other specialists and help you make informed decisions.

If your native language is not English, ask the pharmacy if they can print labels/information in your native language. Some pharmacies can provide drug and label information in multiple languages.

Write what the medication is for on the bottle or lid. This reminder takes the guesswork out of why the drug is needed.

Bring your medications to doctor appointments. Store your medicine and over-the-counter drugs together in a bag. Try to keep them in their original containers, if possible.

Create a medication station. Place pill organizers, pill cutters, crushers, cups, the medication schedule, and other supplies together. Include a list of contact numbers—doctor, pharmacy, poison control, and emergency contacts—for easy access.

Color-code pill bottles. Place color-coded labels on the pill bottles as a reminder of when to take the medication. For example, use yellow for the morning, red for the afternoon, and blue for bedtime.

Take medication with daily events. For example, take morning medication with breakfast and afternoon medication with dinner. Coordination makes it easier to remember.

Refill the pill dispenser at the same time each week. Establish a routine so medication is ready to take when it's time.

Pack enough medications when on the go. When leaving the house, pack enough medication to last the entire trip.

WHAT TO ASK THE DOCTOR

- What is this medication for?

- What are the side effects?

- How do we know if the medicine is helping?

- How long will my loved one need to be on this medication?

- When is the best time to take this?

- Is there anything my loved one needs to avoid or do while taking this?

- What should we do if they miss a dose?

WHAT TO ASK THE PHARMACIST

- Can this medication be crushed?

- Can this be taken with the other medicines? What do we need to know about any possible drug interactions?

- Is there financial assistance we can get for this medication?

HOW ARE YOU DOING?

Helping your loved one manage their medication can be challenging. Short-term memory loss can make it difficult for your loved one to remember when to take their meds. The key to success is being organized and developing a system. A routine will reduce the stress on you and your loved one. Pill organizers, reminders, alarms, and charts can help keep everyone organized. Apps can help track when medications are taken.

At some point, your loved one may refuse to take their medications. Denial, lack of knowledge, or cognitive deficits can contribute to their refusal. This can be stressful. Try to understand why they are resistant. And when you start to lose your patience, it's okay to step away for a few minutes and take a break.

Remember to use your people resources. In chapter 2, we talked about building a healthcare team. When you feel stressed or overwhelmed, that's the perfect time to tap into other members of your team. Get them involved. It's okay if you need help—this is a team effort.

CHAPTER 5

COMMON BEHAVIORAL AND PHYSICAL CHANGES

Simon

Simon pushed Ellen's wheelchair between the rows of tables. Easels and canvases sat on the tabletops along with paint, paintbrushes, palettes, and red plastic cups half-filled with water.

"Where do you want to sit?" he asked his wife.

"In the front, of course," Ellen replied excitedly. Simon noticed that his wife's words still had a soft slur when she got excited. Most people wouldn't hear it, but Simon could tell. Ellen had a stroke about five years ago. Her stroke had left the entire left side of her body paralyzed, and she had difficulty speaking. Her speech had improved with rehab, but there was no improvement to her arm and leg.

Simon wheeled Ellen to the front row, directly in front of the painting instructor. He didn't understand this whole "Paint Night" thing, but Ellen was so excited when she heard about it that he couldn't say no to her. Simon wasn't the artistic type, and, given the choice, he would rather stay home. But Simon loved his wife, and this was something she wanted to do. So here he was, feeling completely out of place.

Simon helped Ellen get set up. He placed all the paint, brushes, and water cup on her right side for easy access. He moved the easel closer so she could reach it from her wheelchair. Then he got settled in front of the easel next to her, with supplies for himself. He had promised Ellen he would try it, too.

Two hours later, Simon had to admit, this Paint Night thing wasn't so bad. His painting wasn't completely horrible—you could identify the tree and mountain scene in the background.

"How's my painting?" he turned to his wife.

"It looks pretty good! This was so much fun!" Ellen exclaimed. Simon looked at his wife's eyes, shining with joy. She looked so beautiful, his heart ached at the sight of her.

"So was it worth it, like I said?" she asked him.

"Yes," Simon replied, gazing at Ellen's megawatt smile. "It was totally worth it."

ANXIETY

A stroke is a life-changing event. It changes the way a person feels, thinks, and moves. Worrying about the future is natural. Everyone needs security, safety, and meaningful relationships. When we fear that our needs aren't going to be met, we worry. Stress can build as your loved one feels worried about responsibilities, work, relationships, and finances. About 25 percent of stroke survivors will experience moderate to severe anxiety.

Your loved one may have feelings of anxiousness for no particular reason or may have anxiety that doesn't go away after a stressful situation. Anxiety is more than just feeling stressed. It is a severe condition that can make it difficult for someone to cope from day to day.

All of this said, anxiety is treatable. If feelings of anxiety don't go away after two weeks, it may be time to see a doctor. The doctor can work to develop a treatment plan that works with your loved one's personal situation, needs, and preferences. This may involve medication or cognitive behavioral therapy and psychological treatments to cope with anxiety.

WHAT TO SAY WHEN YOUR LOVED ONE IS ANXIOUS

"It's okay to be worried. Can you tell me what's bothering you?"
Encourage your loved one to share their worries so you can work through them together.

"You're not alone. I am here for you." Sometimes your loved one needs reassurance that they are safe and secure. You are care partners. Remind them that they don't have to walk this journey alone.

"How can I help you?" Many stroke survivors are worried about becoming a burden. Asking them how you can help may relieve their anxiety of having to ask. Encourage your loved one to take you up on your offer.

WHAT TO DO ABOUT ANXIETY

- **Keep them busy.** Exercise and daily activities will occupy your loved one and divert their thoughts away from worrying. Just about any activity can be adapted for a stroke survivor. The occupational therapist is a great resource to show them how to adapt their hobbies to be one-handed if necessary. A few suggestions:

  - Cooking: Do an internet search for adaptive devices if needed.

  - Singing: Great for someone with speech issues.

  - Puzzles

  - Painting or drawing: Paint by number can be a good place to start.

  - Loom knitting: They can hold down the loom with the affected hand and knit with the other.

  - Adult coloring books

  - Games: Chess, bingo, dominoes, mah-jongg, etc.

  - Computer games: Games that only require a mouse to play include Civilization VI and The Sims.

- Mobile apps: There are apps to help aphasic stroke survivors using games. Any strategy-type game will keep their brain active and promote recovery.

- Writing: The app Dragon Dictation can help.

- **Connect with nature.** Spending time outside is great for reducing stress and anxiety. Exposure to nature makes you feel better emotionally. Try going to the park, starting a garden together, or even bringing nature indoors by placing flowers or plants around the house.

- **Laugh.** Laughing makes people feel good and drives away upsetting emotions. Revisit old stories. Watch a new sitcom together or take your loved one to a comedy club. Hold a dad joke contest and see who can tell the stupidest jokes.

- **Practice deep breathing exercises.** You can do this together to reduce stress. Place your hand over your belly button and relax your stomach muscles. Inhale slowly through your nose for a count of five, then exhale slowly through your mouth for another count of five. Concentrate on the way your stomach moves up and down. Keep breathing this way until you are both relaxed.

- **Spend time doing things they love.** Redirect your loved one's attention by doing things they love, such as hobbies or spending time with friends and family. If they don't have hobbies, try some of the activities listed above.

WHAT TO ASK THE DOCTOR ABOUT ANXIETY

- What are the treatment options for anxiety?

- What kind of therapy is available?

- What lifestyle changes can we make?

- After treatment, when can my loved one expect to feel better?

- How likely is it that the anxiety will return?

COGNITIVE CHANGES

Cognitive changes can occur in different ways, such as short- or long-term memory impairment, loss of emotional control, altered information processing, and visual changes. These are changes that not everyone can see but may still have a significant impact on your loved one's ability to function.

Memory loss may be mild or severe. Some examples of short-term memory loss include the inability to follow a conversation or forgetting where something is located. This can pose a safety hazard if your loved one forgets that the stove is on or can't remember how to make it back home. Long-term memory loss can wipe large portions of your loved one's life from their mind. Your loved one may forget who people are or forget key life events.

Stroke survivors have often told me it takes them longer to think about or process situations after their stroke. This is common, since the brain is trying to heal from the injury. For stroke survivors with more severe symptoms, the inability to problem-solve or make decisions can influence their daily life. If your loved one exhibits poor judgment, they may require close supervision.

Managing emotions can be another challenge. Mood swings or poor impulse control may affect your loved one. Some stroke survivors may suffer from an emotional expression disorder called "pseudo-bulbar affect" (PBA). This disorder causes sudden, uncontrollable, and inappropriate laughing or crying. These emotional outbursts may occur even without a trigger. Stroke survivors with PBA experience emotions normally but occasionally express inappropriate or exaggerated feelings. Because PBA can cause bouts of crying, it may be confused with depression. It is essential to get the proper diagnosis so your loved one can get the appropriate treatment.

Another cognitive change is spatial inattention or neglect, in which the stroke survivor doesn't pay attention to the side of their body affected by the stroke. Your loved one may eat only the food on the right side of their plate because that's all they see, or they may behave like one side of their body does not exist at all.

Visual systems may also be affected by a stroke. Blind spots in your loved one's vision can make tasks such as reading difficult. Tunnel

WHAT TO SAY ABOUT
COGNITIVE CHANGES

"It's okay. Take your time." Stroke survivors suffering from memory loss may experience confusion and agitation. Make eye contact and speak directly to them at a calm and regular rate of speed. Allow them plenty of time to respond.

"Come sit down." Break down tasks and questions into simple terms. Instead of saying, "Would you like to sit on the couch and watch TV?" use smaller sentences such as "Come here" or "Let's watch TV."

WHAT TO DO ABOUT
COGNITIVE CHANGES

Know what's "normal." Explain what your loved one's "new normal" behavior is to your family and friends. It will also help you identify when something is "different," possibly signaling the onset of another stroke.

Get a diagnosis. It is easy to confuse one type of mood swing or cognitive deficit for another. The doctor will be able to diagnose the problem and recommend treatment options.

Place things in their visual field. For stroke survivors who have vision loss or neglect, place items within easy reach in their field of vision. They won't touch their snack if they don't know it's there.

WHAT TO ASK THE DOCTOR
ABOUT COGNITIVE CHANGES

- What kind of treatment is available for this cognitive impairment?

- What non-drug treatment is available?

- Are there coping strategies we can use?

vision or large black spots in their visual field can cause your loved one to seemingly ignore people because they can't see them, or to trip because they don't see an object in their blind spot. Rehabilitation therapy for vision changes involves learning coping techniques, such as scanning or using adaptive tools to compensate for vision loss.

COMMUNICATION

Some stroke survivors may experience difficulty communicating or speaking. An inability to communicate can be isolating for your loved one—imagine being unable to communicate with your family or understand what they are saying to you. By understanding the different communication barriers, you and your loved one can begin to develop strategies for communication.

"Dysarthria" is a speech disorder that causes difficulty saying words. Your loved one's speech may seem slow, slurred, or mumbled. Damage to the part of the brain that controls the lips and tongue muscles may cause your loved one to have difficulty articulating or forming their words. They may also have impaired breath control that changes how their speech sounds.

The inability to communicate is known as "aphasia." It's more common in left-sided strokes. Aphasia involves impairment in four areas:

Spoken language comprehension (receptive aphasia): difficulty understanding what is spoken to them. This is the most challenging type.

Spoken language expression (expressive aphasia): difficulty speaking or finding the right words to say

Reading comprehension: difficulty understanding what they are reading

Written expression: difficulty communicating via writing

Communication strategies for aphasia need to be tailored to the stroke survivor's specific impairment. Work with the speech therapist to develop communication strategies for you and your loved one. Although a stroke survivor may have difficulty communicating, they still

WHAT TO SAY WHEN YOUR LOVED ONE HAS COMMUNICATION DIFFICULTY

"Take your time. I'll wait." Stroke survivors with expressive aphasia or dysarthria can understand you. They only need more time to communicate. Finishing their sentences for them can increase their frustration and resentment.

"Do you want coffee or tea?" Avoid asking open-ended questions. Your loved one may struggle with answering questions. Use questions with a multiple choice or yes/no answer.

WHAT TO DO TO SUPPORT COMMUNICATION

Use eye contact. Avoiding eye contact can be upsetting and hurtful. Stroke survivors deserve the same respect as everyone else.

Use a communication board. Use a picture board or tablet to assist in communication. There are printable aphasia communication boards available online—see the Communication resources section on page 158.

Use multiple forms of communication. Would a video call be more effective so your loved one can see facial expressions and gestures? Would it help for them to have something to write on, like a pad or notebook?

Repeat yourself. When your loved one has trouble understanding you, break things down into smaller steps. Their brain may take more time to process what you are saying.

Don't pretend to understand when you don't. Help your loved one express what they want you to understand. It's more productive for both parties if you understand what they want you to know.

Resist the urge to correct your loved one. It's important to give your loved one the same respect as always, especially when they are trying to build their confidence in communication.

have thoughts and emotions. To a stroke survivor struggling to communicate, it can be frightening when no one understands you or you don't understand what they are saying. Like someone visiting a foreign country who doesn't know the native language, they need to train their brain to learn the "new" language.

DEPRESSION

Stroke survivors are at high risk for developing depression as a result of loss of function and independence. Biochemical changes in the brain can also cause depression. The injury from a stroke may make it challenging to feel positive emotions. Depression is more common in the first year, and one in three people will experience depression within the first five years after a stroke.

After their stroke, your loved one may feel sad or empty and lose interest in things they previously enjoyed doing. They may feel alone or isolated, and find it difficult to concentrate, make decisions, or solve problems. Your loved one may lack energy, sleep more than usual, or have difficulty sleeping. Loss of appetite or changes in weight can be symptoms of depression. Thoughts of death, suicide, or suicide attempts are hazardous and should be taken seriously. The National Suicide Prevention Lifeline is 1-800-273-TALK (8255). This toll-free number will connect you with a trained worker at a local crisis center who will provide confidential support for people experiencing emotional distress or suicidal thoughts.

It is vital to watch for signs of depression so it can be addressed before it hinders recovery. Depression can reduce your loved one's motivation and slow the rehabilitation process. If symptoms persist for more than two weeks, it may be time to see the doctor. Depression is treatable, and a good psychiatrist or psychologist can help. Antidepressants may be prescribed by a doctor. Psychological treatments, such as cognitive behavioral therapy or interpersonal therapy, may also be recommended.

WHAT TO SAY ABOUT DEPRESSION

"I know you feel bad. I'm here to talk when you're ready."
Acknowledge your loved one's feelings and reassure them that you
are there for them. Your loved one may not want to talk right away, but
knowing you're there for them can help them feel supported.

"How are you coping today?" Depression is a medical condition and
should not be treated as a weakness or flaw. Asking about and showing
your support for their depression can help your loved one open up to
you and encourage them to stick to the treatment plan.

"You are important to me because . . ." When someone is depressed,
they may not feel loved or wanted. Telling them why you need them
and love having them in your life can be comforting.

"Can you help me?" Asking for help from your loved one can return
a sense of normalcy and purpose. They will appreciate feeling useful,
whether by being asked for their advice or just listening to you.

WHAT TO DO ABOUT DEPRESSION

Provide opportunities to serve others. Helping others can give your
loved one a sense of purpose and distract them from thinking about
their problems. Can they welcome new members to the church? Can
their hobby help others?

Set goals. Start by setting small, achievable goals together that will give
your loved one a sense of accomplishment, such as setting the table or
doing the dishes. Gradually work up to more challenging goals.

Stay social. Low levels of social support have been linked to depression. Expand your loved one's social circle by involving family and
friends or helping them join a stroke support group.

Restore personal independence. Encourage your loved one to do as
many tasks as they can.

Have fun. Do things your loved one enjoys, even if it feels like a chore.
Your loved one is relearning how to enjoy life.

WHAT TO ASK THE DOCTOR

- How can depression affect stroke recovery?

- Can this depression be treated with psychotherapy, medication, or both?

- How might medications for depression affect other medications my loved one is taking?

- Can other health conditions be contributing to their depression?

- What should I do if my loved one has thoughts of suicide or hurting themself?

FATIGUE

Everyone gets tired once in a while. Fatigue is a common symptom after a stroke and is different from normal tiredness. Post-stroke fatigue doesn't seem to get better with rest and isn't always due to recent activity. There are multiple studies regarding post-stroke fatigue. These studies have shown that fatigue is not related to the type of stroke someone has. Fatigue can be tough on your loved one, and sometimes it can be challenging for them to understand how tired they are.

Many factors could be contributing to your loved one's feelings of fatigue. They may feel tired due to the physical and mental exertion of their rehabilitation exercises. Muscle weakness in affected limbs could use up more energy. Your loved one may be using energy in different ways to compensate for a new disability. Emotional changes like anxiety or depression can contribute to fatigue. Sleep apnea (interrupted breathing), insomnia, joint pain, or muscle stiffness can also make it difficult to sleep. Some medications may have side effects that cause fatigue.

WHAT TO SAY ABOUT FATIGUE

"Are you getting tired?" Ask your loved one if they are getting tired. Sometimes fatigue is not obvious.

"I can see how tired you are. Tell me how you are feeling." Understanding how your loved one is affected can help you and them manage post-stroke fatigue.

WHAT TO DO ABOUT FATIGUE

Manage other draining emotional factors. Anxiety and depression are often linked to fatigue. If your loved one spends less energy struggling with their emotions, there will be more energy left over for rehabilitation.

Pace yourselves. Spread out activities throughout the day or week. Allow your loved one to take rest breaks before they feel too tired.

Know their limits. Keep a diary on how much activity your loved one can do before they get tired. How many rest breaks do they need in between activities? Keep an eye on them at social gatherings so you can see when they seem to be getting tired.

Do one thing at a time. Multitasking can drain energy. Take it slow and focus on one activity at a time.

Wind down for bed. Start a wind-down routine in the early evening to help establish a manageable bedtime routine and ensure that your loved one gets plenty of rest.

WHAT TO ASK THE DOCTOR

- Can any of the medications my loved one is taking cause fatigue?
- What can we do to improve energy levels at home?

PAIN

About 30 percent of stroke survivors experience pain. Stroke pain is more likely to occur in right-sided strokes. Your loved one may describe the pain as aching, burning, or prickling. It can affect the arms, legs, trunk, or even half of their body. It may be described as constant with an occasional stabbing pain. This pain can be affected by changes in temperature or movement and can get worse over time.

Muscle aches and spasticity (involuntary muscle contractions) can be a source of pain. Weakened muscles caused by paralysis on one side are prone to spasms, which may be painful. Spasticity can lead to muscles being permanently shortened. The joints become stiff, so they can't move anymore, leading to contractures (see page 38). Spasticity can become worse in the affected limb and cause pain.

Some stroke survivors may also develop central post-stroke pain (CPSP). This happens if a stroke survivor suffers a stroke in the portion of the brain that interprets pain. Stroke survivors with CPSP may also experience numbness and tingling (pins and needles) in the areas affected by the pain. The pain usually occurs in the side of the body that was affected by the stroke.

Treatment for typical post-stroke pain, which is different than CPSP, can include over-the-counter or prescribed pain medication. For stroke survivors who experience CPSP, pain medication alone may not be effective and they may require additional treatment, such as anti-convulsants, antidepressants, or surgical intervention to manage the pain. Passive range of motion exercises (see page 71) can help keep muscles stretched and prevent contractures. Using splints and braces can help maintain proper body positioning.

WHAT TO SAY ABOUT PAIN

"Are you in pain? Can you show me where?" Don't be afraid to ask your loved one if they are in pain. They may be unable to tell you without assistance.

"Can you rate your pain on a scale of 1 to 10?" Ask your loved one to rate their level of pain. Their response will help you with pain management, and you can provide valuable feedback to their doctor and healthcare team. For stroke survivors who cannot speak, ask them to rate their pain using the Wong-Baker FACES Pain Rating Scale (see Communication resources, page 158) and ask them to point to a face to describe their pain.

WHAT TO DO ABOUT PAIN

Believe them when they say they are in pain. Nothing is more frustrating than someone who doesn't believe you when you are hurting. Research shows that most people do not exaggerate pain just to get sympathy.

Look for nonverbal cues for pain. Be on the lookout for nonverbal cues, such as facial grimacing, grunting, or unwillingness to perform a particular movement. These could be indicators of pain.

Avoid pulling on the shoulder of an affected arm. Be mindful of an affected shoulder when repositioning your loved one. Pulling on the arm or shoulder too hard may cause pain.

Gently massage affected limbs. Fluids may pool in affected limbs due to gravity. Gently massage arms and legs, using long, slow strokes going toward the heart, to help keep their limbs from getting swollen and painful.

Elevate the affected hand. Stroke survivors who have complete paralysis of their arm may develop a swollen hand as the hand hangs downward. Supporting the affected hand with a pillow or cushion can help.

PARALYSIS

Paralysis or loss of sensation is the most common outcome of stroke and can come in many forms. The severity of the paralysis depends on the extent of brain injury. The motor functions of the brain are on the right and left side, at about ear level. Suffering from a stroke in those regions will result in paralysis. Strokes in the posterior (back) of the brain will not exhibit paralysis, but typically result in vision, balance, and coordination deficits, which is where those functions are governed. Most stroke survivors will experience paralysis to some degree immediately following their stroke. Most rehabilitation therapy is focused on paralysis treatment and restoring a stroke survivor to their optimal level of function.

Paralysis may be mild, such as weakness in a hand or leg. Your loved one may have a loss in grip strength or feel numbness in their hand. A stroke survivor once told me, "It's weird; it's like my hand isn't my hand anymore. I can move it, but it feels like someone else's hand." Mild weakness in the leg can cause balance issues and put your loved one at risk for falls. Your loved one may be less coordinated or slower to perform specific tasks.

In severe strokes, a stroke survivor may have "hemiplegia"—complete paralysis of one side of their body. Proper positioning becomes essential so your loved one doesn't develop pressure sores, or bedsores. As their weight is distributed on a bed or chair, bony areas will press on the skin. Prolonged pressure on the skin will cause the skin to break down and sores to develop. Common areas of pressure sores are the buttocks, hips, between the knees, and on the heels. Repositioning your loved one frequently (about every two hours if you can) will help prevent sores and make your loved one more comfortable.

You may notice that your loved one's joints become stiff on their affected arm or leg. Joints that go unused become stiff and lose their flexibility, a condition known as "contracture." Passive range of motion exercises can help keep the joints flexible. These exercises involve gently moving and bending the affected limb at each joint at least 10 times. These exercises can be done once a day, or more often if possible. Splints and orthotics can help support joints and prevent contractures. The physical therapist can develop an exercise plan to perform at home that will help keep joints flexible and mobile.

WHAT TO SAY ABOUT PARALYSIS

"What can I move for you?" Ask your loved one if anything can be moved to increase their comfort, such as a body part, a snack, or the TV remote.

"Are you comfortable?" What is comfortable to you may not be comfortable for them. Your loved one will appreciate being asked.

WHAT TO DO ABOUT PARALYSIS

Reposition often. I cannot stress this enough. Whether it is repositioning your loved one's body or helping them perform passive range of motion exercises, this is important. Pressure sores are painful, and contractures can cause pain and hinder your loved one's rehabilitation efforts.

Perform a skin check. Check your loved one's skin regularly for signs of redness or a break in the skin. Pay particular attention to areas where their body weight could be placing pressure.

If it looks uncomfortable, it probably is. If your loved one is positioned in a way that looks uncomfortable to you, it probably is. Don't be afraid to offer to change their body position.

Use proper body mechanics. Don't hurt yourself moving your loved one around. Ask the physical therapist for techniques to minimize the strain on your own body.

WHAT TO ASK THE DOCTOR ABOUT PARALYSIS

- What type of rehabilitation therapy is needed?

- What exercises can we do to help with the paralysis?

- Are there any assistive devices we can use?

- Are there any splints or orthotics that can help?

SEIZURES

Stroke survivors are at an increased risk for seizures. Scar tissue forms in the injured portions of their brain and alters the electrical activity. When electrical pathways are disrupted, this can cause seizures. Stroke survivors who have had hemorrhagic (bleeding) strokes are more likely to have seizures. The more severe the stroke, the greater the risk of seizure. The first 30 days post-stroke carry the highest risk for seizures.

There are more than 40 different types of seizures, and some are more dangerous than others. Seizures can be divided into two main categories: focal onset seizures and generalized seizures. Focal onset seizures start in a single point of the brain. This may only start with twitching in one part of the body, like their face or arm. As the seizure progresses, your loved one may zone out or stare into space. They may not remember anything unusual happening during the episode. In some focal seizures, a person can stay aware or awake while it is happening.

Generalized seizures start in multiple points of the brain all at once and can affect the entire body. This type of seizure is the most well-known and can be scary to watch. A generalized seizure is known as a "grand mal" or "tonic-clonic" seizure, and it follows a sequence of events:

Unresponsiveness: The person doesn't react when you shake them or call their name. They may collapse suddenly.

Tonic phase: The person becomes as stiff as a board, as their muscles clench for a few seconds.

Clonic phase: The body undergoes convulsions that jerk their body around. This can last a few seconds or several minutes.

Post-ictal state: This period of confusion, drowsiness, or disorientation follows a seizure. They may experience a temporary weakness or paralysis in their limbs, known as "Todd's paralysis."

Seizures do not usually need medical attention. The Centers for Disease Control and Prevention (CDC) recommends calling 911 if one or more of the following are true:

- This is their first seizure.

- The person has difficulty waking or breathing after the seizure.

- The seizure lasts more than five minutes.

- The person experiences another seizure soon after the first one.

- The person injures themselves during the seizure.

- The seizure happened in water.

- The person has a health condition, such as heart disease or diabetes, or is pregnant.

Seizures, whatever the type, can be treated with antiseizure medication. Your doctor can work with you on the best combination of drugs to treat seizures for your loved one. Some diets high in fat and low in carbohydrates, such as a ketogenic diet, can reduce the frequency of seizures. Ask your doctor or dietitian if changes in your loved one's diet could help.

HOW ARE YOU DOING?

There was a lot of content here because your loved one could have any combination of issues we've discussed. I hope that reading this has given you a better idea of what to expect and what you can do to help your loved one.

Having a stroke fundamentally changes someone. It can change how your loved one processes information and emotions, how they communicate, and how they move through the world. It changes the way they live life, and the struggle for most stroke survivors is learning how to live in a meaningful way again.

As their care partner, you walk this path with your loved one. Together, you navigate unfamiliar territory. I hope this chapter gave you a better understanding of their struggles.

WHAT TO SAY ABOUT SEIZURES

"You just had a seizure. What did you feel just before it happened?"
Keeping a seizure diary can help track when seizures happen and identify potential triggers.

WHAT TO DO ABOUT SEIZURES

If your loved one is experiencing a seizure:

- Keep other people out of the way.

- Don't stop your loved one's movements unless they are in danger.

- Roll your loved one on their side to prevent vomiting and choking.

- Cushion your loved one's head and loosen any clothing around their neck.

- Avoid putting anything in your loved one's mouth.

- Move sharp or solid objects out of the way, so your loved one doesn't hit them during during their seizure.

- Keep track of how long the seizure lasts and what symptoms occurred before their seizure so you can inform emergency personnel.

- Stay with your loved one until their seizure ends. If this is a first seizure OR the seizure persists longer than five minutes, call 911.

WHAT TO ASK THE DOCTOR ABOUT SEIZURES

- What tests are needed to evaluate seizure activity?

- What medications will we need to control seizures?

- Is there any food that we can avoid to improve seizure control?

- Are there other treatments for seizures that are right for my loved one?

The effects of stroke vary. Your loved one may have mild deficits and require minimal assistance, or they might have severe deficits that require a lot of help. Taking care of a stroke survivor can require physical exertion that taxes your body. Get lessons in proper body mechanics from the physical therapist. The saying "Lift with your knees, not with your back" is relevant and a good place to start. The physical therapist will help you learn how to use your own body weight to your advantage and offer other techniques to help your move your loved one safely. These lessons can keep you from hurting yourself.

Combat the physical toll by taking time to decompress and take care of your body. Place a heated wrap around your shoulders for 15 to 30 minutes. Online stores sell microwavable or electric heating pads for a reasonable price. Use this pad to relax the tension in your neck and shoulders. You can also try placing a tennis ball between your back and the wall. Press and hold the ball for a few seconds to relieve tension in your shoulders and back.

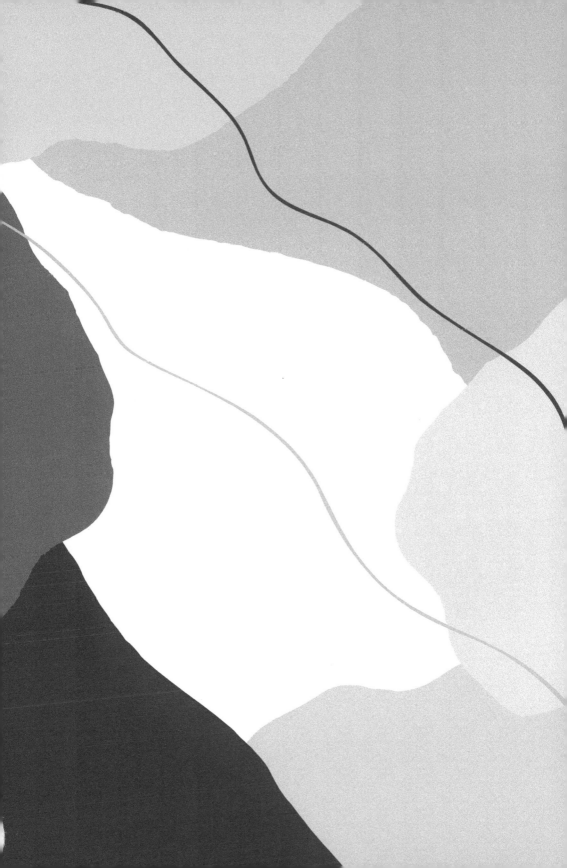

CHAPTER 6

COMMON DAILY LIVING CHANGES

Ana

"Ana, I need to go to the bathroom," her grandmother told her. Ana knelt in front of her grandmother's armchair. She placed her hands on Grandma's hips and gently helped her move her bottom to the edge of the chair. Then she repositioned the walker so it was in front of the armchair. Her grandmother grasped the sides of the walker as leverage and pulled herself out of the chair. Grandma pushed the walker forward and started to make her way to the bathroom, her left foot dragging slightly behind. Ana walked slightly behind her and watched for any indication that her grandmother was off balance.

In the bathroom, Ana helped Grandma position herself on the raised toilet seat. She was glad Grandma wore a dress today because it made helping her with her underwear easier. She took the bidet hand sprayer off the wall next to the toilet and handed it to her grandmother. Then she moved the walker nearby.

"I'll check on you in a few minutes," she told Grandma as she closed the bathroom door. "Don't get up without me."

"Okay," her grandmother assured her.

Ana headed back to the kitchen table to clean up from breakfast. Grandma lived with Ana's aunt, who was her primary caregiver. But today, Ana was taking her turn relieving her aunt so her aunt could have a break. Ever since Grandma's stroke two years ago, Ana came over every other Saturday to help.

Ana noticed how many things in the house had changed. Gone were all the rugs on the floor, furniture was rearranged to create wider spaces, and all the doorknobs were changed to lever handles instead of the old twist knobs. Her aunt had installed handrails next to the toilet and tub. Grandma's shower chair dominated the middle of the tub, along with a bright yellow non-skid rug. The insurance company provided her with a hospital bed that could be raised and lowered.

Ana chuckled as she remembered the ceramic figures that her aunt used to have decorating every table and horizontal surface. As a child, Ana wasn't allowed to touch the expensive figures for fear of breaking them. Those were gone now, probably stored in boxes in the garage.

Ana cleared the table and washed the breakfast dishes. Grandma's plate had a suction cup bottom and her utensils had fat handles that made them easier to grip. Her grandmother only drank from cups with handles and spill guards now. Ana dried her hands on the dish towel. "Time to check on Grandma," she said to herself, and headed back to the bathroom.

SAFETY AT HOME

There's no place like home, and this is especially true after a hospital or rehab stay. Your loved one will be eager to come home to a familiar space. But home can take adjusting to, also. Strokes can change the way your loved one moves about their home and performs tasks. These changes can be short-term or permanent. By making some simple adjustments to the home, you will increase safety and navigability for your loved one to ease back into their home life.

Falling is a common risk among stroke survivors and can be very dangerous. Limited mobility, balance and vision changes, and the risk of post-stroke seizures make them prone to falling. By performing a home assessment and making some home modifications, you can help reduce the risk of falling:

- Make sure pathways around the house are clear of any clutter that could cause your loved one to trip.

- Place non-skid rubber backings on any floor rugs, or consider removing rugs completely from the home.

- Station a commode at the bedside to eliminate the need to make a trip to the bathroom at night.

- Place handrails in the bathroom and near stairs or steps to make them easier to navigate.

- If possible, install ramps where steps are.

If your loved one falls and experiences bruising, bleeding, or pain, call 911 or go to the closest emergency room. Falling while taking a blood thinner can result in internal bleeding that may not be visible. Seek emergency services right away if your loved one falls while taking a blood thinner medication (anything other than aspirin). Tell emergency personnel what blood thinner medication your loved one is on, as they may be able to reverse any bleeding in the hospital.

Take advantage of technology when implementing safety strategies in the home. Set up a medical alert system with a wearable emergency medical button. If your loved one is amenable to it, consider installing cameras to monitor their safety in the common areas of the home. This can be useful for long-distance caregivers who are unable to be at their loved one's side at all times. Not all stroke survivors will be comfortable with this and may see it as an invasion of privacy, so it's important to be sensitive to their concerns.

DOCTORS' APPOINTMENTS

For stroke survivors, caregivers must often coordinate treatments among multiple specialists or rehabilitation therapists, and multiple doctors' visits. A continuum of follow-up care is essential for stroke recovery and the prevention of recurrent strokes.

In all of this, you may need to advocate for your loved one. Don't assume that the primary care physician and the specialists are communicating regularly. The physician and the specialist may not have access to each other's medical records. Check if a medical records release form can be filled out for each clinic, so they can share medical information. One doctor may assume the other doctor will order a medication or referral, and things may be lost or overlooked due to miscommunication between the two clinics.

One obstacle that caregivers often face is resistance by their loved one to go to their follow-up appointments. If your loved one is feeling

WHAT TO SAY ABOUT SAFETY

"Remember not to hold onto the chairs while walking." Furniture can slide and throw your loved one off balance. Encourage them to use their assistive device, such as a cane or walker, instead.

"Take your time; there's no rush." Encourage your loved one to take their time moving around to prevent falls and injuries.

"Are you ready to come out of the bathroom?" If your loved one is taking more time than usual in the bathroom, don't be afraid to check on them. They may need help with toileting or bathing, or may have fallen and need immediate assistance.

WHAT TO DO TO KEEP YOUR LOVED ONE SAFE

Don't lock the bathroom door. Encourage your loved one not to lock the bathroom door when they are using it, or, if they agree, remove the lock on the door. Make it a house rule that a closed bathroom door indicates the need for privacy. If your loved one falls or is otherwise in need of assistance, you need to be able to open the door right away without the lock in the way. (Note: This is a good rule for public bathrooms, as well. Tell them not to lock it and you'll stand guard outside the door.)

Install lever handles. Lever handles on doors and faucets are easier to operate than a knob you have to twist.

Use pump bottles. Putting liquids like soap, shampoo, conditioner, lotion, and mouthwash in pump bottles can make it easier for your loved one to dispense the contents.

Buy toothpaste with flip-top caps. Flip-top caps are easier to open than screw-on caps.

Check the hot water. Consider resetting the hot water heater temperature to a lower setting if your loved one lives alone and has difficulty with regulating the water temperature.

Wear proper footwear. Non-skid, flat, wide-toed shoes can increase your loved one's stability. Avoid house slippers or flip-flops that can slide off their feet. Use socks with non-skid bottoms and ensure they fit properly so they don't slide off their feet.

Widen the space. Widen the spaces between furniture. At least a 32-inch clearance is needed to accommodate a wheelchair. If it helps, consider removing unnecessary doors between rooms.

Encourage use of walker brakes. When they are getting up to use their walker, or going down a step to their walker, encourage them to use the brakes if their walker is equipped, so the walker doesn't move.

Store one walker upstairs and another downstairs. This will minimize the need to move the walker between the two floors.

Make phones accessible. Place cordless phones in a handy location in every room of the house. If your loved one is able to use a cell phone, consider using a cell phone lanyard with a breakaway clasp that they can wear around their neck for easy access.

Hide wires. Keep wires and cords behind furniture and out of your loved one's path.

Keep things within easy reach. Easy access to food, cooking supplies, clothes, and other essentials is vital for stroke survivors. Move difficult-to-access items to lower shelves or drawers. Consider open shelving, baskets for storage, or a lazy Susan to increase access. Labeling food and other items can help stroke survivors with memory problems.

WHAT TO ASK THE DOCTOR ABOUT SAFETY

- What exercises can we do to build leg strength and balance?

- What can we do to prevent falls?

- Do you have any tips on how to make things safer?

better, they may not see a reason to go, or they might feel that they are a burden for going. Talk to your loved one and allow them to express their concerns. Reassure them you are care partners and address their concerns. Encourage them to stay consistent with their follow-up care.

EATING AND NUTRITION

It can be a challenge to ensure that your loved one is getting proper nutrition after a stroke. Eating can be difficult due to a weakness of the hand or arm that causes problems using utensils. Your loved one may need some adaptive devices to help them eat, such as large handles on utensils or rubber pads to keep plates from sliding.

A heart-healthy diet is recommended for stroke survivors. This means a diet low in salt and cholesterol and high in fiber to help prevent another stroke. Too much salt can cause water retention, which increases blood pressure. A low-cholesterol diet will reduce the buildup of plaque in the blood vessels. Eating a high-fiber diet can reduce cholesterol and control blood sugar levels. Stroke survivors may be prone to constipation due to reduced mobility, so a high-fiber diet has the added bonus of promoting bowel regularity.

Your loved one may have a decreased appetite or memory loss that causes them to forget to eat or drink. Your best strategy is to prepare food that they like, or food that looks and smells good. Eating small, frequent meals may stimulate their appetite. If your loved one struggles with getting enough nutrition, a dietitian can recommend supplements for them.

We've talked about dysphagia, a condition that causes difficulty swallowing or an uncoordinated swallow. When that happens, food spills into the throat too quickly and can cause coughing or choking. If food or fluid travels down the trachea (windpipe) and into the lungs, it can potentially lead to the lung infection known as pneumonia. For stroke survivors who have dysphagia, it is recommended to eat slowly and use a teaspoon to ensure that food is being consumed in smaller amounts. Avoid using a straw for drinking liquids, as that, too, can cause liquids to be sucked in too quickly and cause choking. Have your loved

WHAT TO SAY ABOUT FOOD

"Let's have dinner at Mary's house!" Eating with other people can stimulate the appetite. Your loved one may eat more if meals are fun and spent socializing with friends and family.

"What would you like to eat this week?" Create a meal plan with your loved one. Provide multiple options to choose from. Encourage them to select foods they enjoy, including snacks and dessert. Choose heart-healthy foods as much as possible.

"Let's get something to drink." Ensure that your loved one has plenty of water to drink. Dehydration can suppress the appetite.

WHAT TO DO ABOUT EATING

Eat nutrient-dense, high-calorie foods first. The best opportunity to get calories and nutrition inside your loved one is at the beginning of the meal, before they lose their appetite or get too tired to eat any more.

Use a large plate. The task of eating seems less daunting when the plate looks less full.

Pack snacks. When you're out with your loved one, take advantage of sudden hunger strikes by having snacks available. Sharing a snack is a great way to spend time together.

Perform oral hygiene regularly. This will prevent mouth sores that may make eating painful or unpleasant.

Check dentures. Ill-fitting dentures are painful and can make eating uncomfortable. Ensure that dentures are properly fitted.

Meal-prep and freeze extras. Make meals that you can freeze ahead of time. This will save you time on days you are too tired or busy to cook.

WHAT TO ASK THE DOCTOR ABOUT NUTRITION

- Are there any diet restrictions we need to follow?

- How do we know my loved one is getting proper nutrition?

- Do any of their medications affect appetite or how food tastes?

- Should my loved one be taking supplements?

Questions to ask if your loved one has a PEG tube:

- How will we know if the PEG tube gets infected?

- How will we know if the tube is blocked? What should we do if that happens?

- What should we do if the tube gets pulled out?

- How are medications, water, and food given through the PEG tube?

- How do we empty the stomach through the tube?

- What are the best ways to hide the PEG tube under clothes?

- What kinds of activities should we avoid?

- Do you have any tips on PEG tube safety?

one sit upright in a chair during their meal and for 30 minutes after—this will aid safe swallowing and digestion.

Dysphagia may cause difficulty chewing and an issue called "pocketing" food. Pocketing food happens as a result of decreased sensation in the mouth and uncoordinated chewing. Food gets trapped in a "pocket" inside the lips, cheeks, and gums. The stroke survivor may not feel the food that falls in those gaps, nor are they able to maneuver the food out of the pocket. If your loved one has been known to pocket food, ask them to open their mouth after their meal and check for food. Ask your loved one to sweep their tongue from side to side to try to dislodge any food, or ask them to do a finger sweep inside their mouth. Consider using a mouth swab or Toothette to help them remove the excess food particles. If that doesn't work, give them some fluid to drink and try to wash it down.

Stroke survivors who have dysphagia may need a modified-texture diet, or "dysphagia diet," to promote safe swallowing. The speech therapist will recommend the texture for food and liquids that best supports safe swallowing. Thickening powder may be added to liquids to get the desired consistency. In 2019, the International Dysphagia Diet Standardisation Initiative (IDDSI) replaced a previously adopted scale called the National Dysphagia Diet (NDD). The new IDDSI guidelines outline clear definitions of diet consistency for food and drink. See the Nutrition resources (page 160) for more information on IDDSI.

Stroke survivors who have completely lost the ability to swallow may need to have a percutaneous endoscopic gastrostomy (PEG) tube inserted. The doctor places a flexible tube through the abdomen and into the stomach. Two small discs along the tube, one on the inside of the stomach and one on the outside of the abdomen close to the skin, keep the PEG tube in position. Marks along the outside of the tube help confirm that it is in the correct position. The PEG tube often has a clamp to seal it and ports on the end through which medication, water, and liquid formula can be given to your loved one. If your loved one comes home with a PEG tube, a nurse will train you and your loved one on the proper care and cleaning of the tube and how to use it to safely deliver medication, food, and water.

FAMILY COMMUNICATOR

The family communicator acts as the primary contact who distributes information to the family. If you are the primary caregiver to your loved one, you are most likely the family communicator as well. As the person who knows the most about the stroke survivor, the primary caregiver is often the natural choice to be the family communicator.

One of the most important duties as family communicator is to be your loved one's advocate. As the champion of their care, it's up to the family communicator to ensure the loved one's needs and desires are expressed to both the healthcare team and the rest of the family. Fulfilling this role requires the family communicator to listen carefully to their loved one's wishes, and do their best to include them in all decisions regarding their care.

As the family member with the most knowledge about the loved one's medical history, the family communicator provides valuable information that assists the healthcare team in decision-making. Keeping track of all the details can be challenging, so see the What to Do to Be a Family Communicator section on page 89 for an outline detailing how to organize a medical information binder.

Other family members rely on the family communicator to provide updates on their loved one. Private social media groups can be an effective tool for sending updates to family members all at once. By posting photos and videos that chronicle your loved one's stroke recovery, you can rally support from close friends and family. Posts don't always have to be about medical issues. Shine the spotlight on fun activities that your loved one engaged in or videos that celebrate successes to keep people engaged in your loved one's care.

PERSONAL HYGIENE

Some stroke survivors need help with personal hygiene. An occupational therapist can help your loved one relearn skills to perform these tasks. The occupational therapist can recommend adaptive equipment to maximize their independence, including:

- Shower chair: Bathing and showering can be made easier with a shower chair so your loved one can sit comfortably while bathing.

- Handheld shower head: This can spray water where it is needed most.

- Grab bars on the wall and non-slip mats on the floor: These can increase safety while bathing.

- A long-handled scrubber: This handy tool makes scrubbing hard-to-reach parts of the body easier.

WHAT TO SAY TO YOUR LOVED ONE

"What's important to you?" As your loved one's advocate, have conversations with them about what is important to their care, activities they enjoy, or even things they dislike. Have this conversation regularly to stay up-to-date on their wishes.

"Let's take a selfie!" Encourage your loved one to make memories with the people they love and preserve those moments for the future.

WHAT TO DO TO BE A FAMILY COMMUNICATOR

A three-ring binder can consolidate and help keep track of your loved one's important information. Include tabs for the following sections. Take the binder with you to any appointments or hospital visits.

Emergency contacts: Include emergency contacts, their relationship to your loved one, and their contact information. Note any special roles that may be assigned to different family members, such as primary caregiver, the person who oversees your loved one's finances, or the person who makes medical decisions when your loved one is unable to make them.

Healthcare team: Include contact information for each member of the healthcare team, including the primary care physician, neurologist, and/or any other specialists and the reason your loved one is seeing them. Include addresses and contact numbers.

Appointments: Store medical appointment cards and documentation for upcoming appointments.

Medical history: Write down any medical diagnoses and when your loved one was diagnosed, such as hypertension (high blood pressure), diabetes, or strokes. Add a section for family medical history for your loved one's parents, grandparents, siblings, aunts, and uncles. Track your loved one's surgical history in this section, and note any surgeries and procedures with the date they occurred. Place photocopies of cards that contain implant information such as pacemakers, stents, or rods and pins. Highlight any metal implants. This is important if your loved one needs a magnetic resonance imaging (MRI) scan. Most metal implants are not safe around an MRI due to the strong magnetic field generated by the machine, and your loved one may not be able to have an MRI safely if they have any metal inside their body.

Medications: At the top of this page, write any allergies that your loved one has. List the medications your loved one is taking. Include any vitamins, supplements, and over-the-counter medications, and their dosages.

Insurance: Include photocopies of your loved one's medical, dental, and vision insurance cards. Include contact numbers for customer service for each insurance provider.

Legal: Store copies of legal documents, such as durable power of attorney, or living wills/advance directives. See chapter 7 for more information about legal documents.

Logs: Store any logs you are using to keep track of your loved one's health information, such as a blood sugar log, blood pressure log, seizure diary, or exercise log.

WHAT TO ASK FAMILY AND FRIENDS

- What's the easiest way to contact you?
- How often would you like updates?
- Would you like to join a private social media group to see updates?

Toileting can be made easier with a few modifications:

- Grab bars next to the toilet: These can make sitting and standing easier and safer.

- A raised toilet seat: This can also make sitting and standing easier.

- Self-assist toilet wiping aids: These are long sticks with grippers that hold the toilet paper.

- Handheld bidet sprayer next to the toilet: This can help your loved one clean themselves thoroughly.

Some stroke survivors will suffer from incontinence or difficulty controlling their bladder and bowel movements. Incontinence can be awkward and embarrassing. Urinary incontinence is more common in stroke survivors. The doctor can help you formulate a plan for managing incontinence, preventing associated skin breakdown, and avoiding urinary tract infections.

RETURNING TO WORK

Many stroke survivors long to return to their pre-stroke way of life. The desire to return to work can be a good source of motivation for working toward rehab goals. With proper care and support, many stroke survivors can return to work.

Whether your loved one is able to return to work depends in part on their deficits, the kind of work they do, and the support their employer can provide. The Americans with Disabilities Act (ADA) requires employers to provide reasonable accommodations for people with disabilities. Returning to work does not necessarily mean that a person will return to the same job or responsibilities. Depending on the nature of the job, your loved one's employer may be able to adjust their previous role or offer another role that is better suited to their current abilities. In some instances, putting your loved one's employer in touch with their occupational therapist can help the employer understand how the stroke impacted your loved one.

WHAT TO SAY ABOUT PERSONAL HYGIENE

"I'm glad you're letting me help you. It helps when we work as a team." Reassure your loved one that you are on their side. They will appreciate not being a burden.

"You take the scrubber, and I'll take the handheld shower head." Care partners working together makes things easier. Encourage your loved one to do as much as they can for themselves.

WHAT TO DO ABOUT HYGIENE

Have them wear the right clothing. Wearing clothing that is easy to put on and take off can help with dressing and toileting.

Establish a toileting routine. Schedule regular bathroom breaks among daily activities to minimize accidents.

Check for incontinence often. Your loved one may not be able to tell you when they have an accident. Prompt cleanup can prevent rashes and skin breakdown.

Coordinate timing for drinking liquids. Drinks such as coffee and tea are natural diuretics and increase the need to urinate. Control when your loved one drinks coffee or tea, and schedule a bathroom break about an hour after they drink.

Prepare the bathroom in advance. Set up the bathroom before bath time or a scheduled bathroom break. Place things you will need close at hand to make the task easier.

Protect their modesty. Preserving modesty can be important to your loved one. Allow some privacy and only uncover your loved one when absolutely necessary. Allow your loved one to wear underwear during bath time if that's most comfortable for them.

Moisturize them. Keeping your loved one's skin soft and supple will reduce the incidence of skin tears and skin breakdown.

Be diligent about oral care. Mouth bacteria can get into the bloodstream and increase the risk of clot formation. Poor oral hygiene has also been linked to an increase risk of aspiration pneumonia in stroke survivors.

Perform regular nail care. Keep your loved one's nails short. Soaking their hands and feet in warm water before you start can help soften their nails and make clipping their nails easier.

WHAT TO ASK THE DOCTOR ABOUT HYGIENE

- Do you have any recommendations for treating incontinence?

- Are there medications that can help with incontinence?

- Are there any ointments or creams we can use to prevent skin breakdown?

- Do you have any recommendations for equipment to help with dressing and personal hygiene?

WHAT TO SAY ABOUT RETURNING TO WORK

"Is returning to work one of your goals?" The American Stroke Association offers some great resources for stroke survivors who are considering returning to work. See the Return to Work resources section (page 161) for more information.

"I know one of your goals is to return to work. Let's make a plan on how to achieve it." Review your loved one's rehab goals and create a plan. The American Stroke Association's Return to Work Goal Setting worksheet (See page 161) is a good place to start.

"You've been working hard at rehab. You are getting closer to your goal of returning to work." They'll appreciate your support and encouragement as they strive for their goal.

WHAT TO DO TO SUPPORT RETURN TO WORK

Keep your loved one's employer in the loop. Speak with their employer's human resources department. They can assist with the process of requesting accommodations and explore how your loved one can return to work.

Sign up early for Social Security benefits. If your loved one is planning to go on disability, start the process right away. Gather all the required documents to minimize delays in the application process. More information on Social Security benefits can be found in chapter 7.

Research employers that hire disabled workers. Some employers hire workers with a variety of deficits. See the Return to Work resources section (page 161) for employer databases.

WHAT TO ASK THE DOCTOR ABOUT WORK

- Is returning to work an option?

- What accommodations may be needed in order for my loved one to return to work?

Some effects of stroke can affect your loved one's ability to work. Fatigue is a common symptom, so your loved one may get tired more easily or frequently. Some stroke survivors find it more effective to return to work gradually and build up their stamina. Part-time hours may be helpful at first, while slowly increasing hours. For some stroke survivors, returning to their current job may not be possible. Stroke survivors who are unable to return to work may find fulfillment in volunteering their time.

SEX AND INTIMACY

Sex is a natural part of healthy intimate relationships. Strokes can impact the lives of couples who are sexually active. Couples should take the process of reintroducing intimacy in the relationship slowly, to give both of them time to adjust to any changes or issues.

The location of the stroke can impact sexual behavior and decrease the level of desire. A stroke may also decrease inhibitions and awareness of socially appropriate behavior. In rare cases, a stroke can increase sex drive and make your loved one hypersexual.

Some couples may worry if having sex is safe. In most cases, having sex does not increase the risk of having another stroke. An increase in breathing and heart rate is normal, and having sex typically uses as much energy as climbing two flights of stairs.

Strokes can decrease sensation and limit mobility. Things might feel different for your loved one. Propping up the weaker side of the body can help if paralysis or muscle weakness are an issue. The more mobile person should consider taking the top position. Experiment with new positions and see what makes you both feel good.

If you and your loved one are having problems resuming intimacy, don't be afraid to seek outside help. A doctor, counselor, or social worker can help address your concerns and provide resources. When you are feeling frustrated, remember there are many ways to express that you care for each other and share intimacy.

STAYING ACTIVE

The physical therapist can help coach you on safe exercises your loved one can do. Daily activities should support physical limitations and promote stroke recovery. For stroke survivors, new guidelines recommend simple activities that slowly build strength and endurance. These can even include performing household chores or walking around the neighborhood. Sitting and standing intermittently can gradually build leg strength. Some exercises can be performed while sitting, such as seated marching or leg extensions.

While physical activity is essential, it's also important to stimulate the mind with cognitive activities and games. Cognitive activities, such as memory boards or puzzles, stimulate neuroplasticity, which is the brain's ability to create new nerve pathways.

There are many online resources for physical and cognitive stroke exercises. A simple internet search can provide many links, examples, and videos for various activities. Searching for "stroke rehab games" can also yield a multitude of games that support stroke recovery.

HOW ARE YOU DOING?

Balancing your loved one's physical, emotional, spiritual, and sexual needs can put a lot of strain on your own well-being. Some of your new responsibilities may be unfamiliar, and it can be overwhelming to think about your to-do list. Stop for a moment, take a deep breath, and remember to tackle one thing at a time.

Your resources for help aren't limited to friends, family, and/or the healthcare team. Your loved one is the other half of your care partnership, and may be able to help as well. Even with limited physical mobility, your loved one can be a willing ear to listen. If they understand your frustrations, they may strive to help you in whatever way they can. Stroke survivors crave a sense of independence, and being able to help, even in some small way, can give them that. Your partnership can grow if there is mutual trust and understanding.

WHAT TO SAY ABOUT INTIMACY

"Let's snuggle." Hugging and cuddling are just as important as having sex. Intimacy through embracing and kissing can convey love just as effectively.

"I love you, and I want to share this with you." Reassuring your loved one that you still want to be intimate can help soothe their apprehensions.

"Does this hurt?" or **"That hurts."** The way you move and feel is different after a stroke. Keep lines of communication open to make sure you're not hurting each other during sex.

"Let's try . . ." If something isn't working well, don't be afraid to try something else. Experiment with different positions, techniques, tools, or toys to see what works best for you and your loved one.

WHAT TO DO ABOUT SEX

Take it slow. After a stroke, there are often emotions, insecurities, or concerns that can hinder intimacy. Make sure you and your loved one are both ready.

Talk openly and honestly about your desires. Speaking honestly about desires, fears, and concerns can help keep you connected and reduce negative emotions such as anger and resentment.

Use the power of touch. Sometimes the best way to communicate intimacy or desire is through touch. Touching, caressing, and hugging can convey feelings of love or desire without the use of words.

Plan it out. Consider the best time to be physically intimate with your loved one. Is it better in the morning when they are well rested and not too tired? Would it be better to try sex before taking blood pressure or antidepressant medication that could reduce desire or prevent an erection?

Set the mood. Prepare candles, pillows and props, or music to set the stage. Keep things such as massage oils or lubricants close at hand.

WHAT TO ASK THE DOCTOR ABOUT SEX

- Is it safe to resume sex?

- Can any of their medications be affecting my loved one's sexual desire?

- Do you have any recommendations to help maintain an erection?

- Do you have any recommendations on how to deal with my loved one's hypersexuality?

In hectic times, you'll need a way to de-stress. Listening to music can help, and music is good for the soul in many ways. Reading for fun isn't always possible when things are really busy, but listening to an audiobook or podcast while on the go is an option. Work isn't such a chore when you're listening to something fun while doing it. Find a topic or music you love, and listen while you're driving, cleaning, or otherwise doing something around the house. Or, if you need that moment to unwind, put some gentle sounds on and just relax.

WHAT TO SAY TO STAY ACTIVE

"Let's get some fresh air and go for a walk." Walking 30 minutes a day three to five times a week can help keep your loved one active. A walk with a destination such as a nearby park or shop can help motivate your loved one and may provide an opportunity to rest (or shop!) before heading back home.

"Let's do some stretches together." Performing stretches and passive range of motion exercises prevents muscle shortening and improves flexibility.

"You've worked hard. Time for a break." Give muscles a chance to rest and recover. Don't let your loved one get so tired that they can't participate in exercise regularly.

WHAT TO DO TO KEEP YOUR LOVED ONE ACTIVE

Minimize bed rest. Unless they are very fatigued, encourage your loved one to spend as much time out of bed as they can, even if it's just sitting in a chair.

Exercise during commercials. Encourage your loved one to take advantage of commercial breaks during television shows and perform some seated exercises.

WHAT TO ASK THE DOCTOR ABOUT EXERCISE

- How much exercise should we be doing?

- What kind of exercise can we do at home?

- What resources do you suggest for stroke exercises?

- Are there any useful videos or instructions you can recommend?

CHAPTER 7

FINANCIAL AND LEGAL DECISIONS

Sam

Sam was worried. His mom's health seemed to be slowly declining, and he knew that they would have to make tough decisions soon. His mom, Iris, had a stroke about eight years ago, leaving her right leg very weak. Iris could get around with a walker without too much help until a couple of months ago, when she suffered a seizure, fell, and broke her left hip. She had a hip replacement, then went to a rehab facility to regain mobility in her hip. Despite rehab, Iris was no longer able to get out of bed. Now that she was in bed all the time, the spark was gone from her eyes, and she just looked tired.

Sam had always taken care of his mom. Iris had lived with him ever since her stroke. Sam had three brothers and a sister, but they were "too busy" or didn't have space to take care of their mother. Their visits were limited to holidays or major family gatherings. Sam didn't like that his siblings were content to let him perform all the caregiving duties but still voiced their opinions on how their mother should be treated.

On the advice of a close friend, Sam called an attorney about setting up his mother's will. The attorney brought up many things that Sam hadn't even thought about, like documents to designate financial and medical decisions. He and his mom had never talked about such things. How could he bring up such issues with his brothers and sister? Inwardly Sam cringed at the thought of holding the conversation, but he knew his mother would want his siblings involved. He was not looking forward to speaking to one opinionated brother in particular, but the lawyer had advised him that it was better to have things clearly documented in the legal paperwork. It would avoid confusion and conflict later, the lawyer told him.

Sam needed to talk to his mother first before anything else. He knocked softly on Iris's open bedroom door before stepping inside. He took a deep breath.

"Hey, Mom," he said. "Can I talk to you about something?"

FINANCES

Stroke survivors and caregivers will need to do a fair amount of financial planning after a stroke. Budgeting for healthcare expenses, medication prescriptions, and extra help may have to be factored in. Your loved one may not be able to manage their finances effectively post-stroke, but assigning someone they trust to oversee finances can help relieve the burden of paying bills and managing their accounts.

Talking about money with your loved one can be difficult. It's scary giving up independence over your money. It can be difficult to balance the need to protect your loved one's finances with their freedom to make decisions. Some initial suggestions include:

Go over finances and bills together. Having the chance to be involved may ease their concerns. Build trust by letting them know where their money is going and making finance decisions together.

Consider setting spending limits on credit cards. This can help curb spending if that becomes an issue.

Set money aside for a "treat yourself" purchase. Concessions like these can help your loved one feel less restricted.

The key to managing the financial side of stroke is applying for financial aid early, since the application process for some benefits can take months. Refer to the Finances resources section (page 158) for more information.

Short-Term Disability (STD)

Short-term disability benefits may provide limited financial support and salary replacement for non-job-related injuries or illnesses. Short-term disability may be offered by an employer or obtained through a licensed disability insurance company. Coverage and payments depend on the policy. Short-term disability benefits can be as short as 30 days and are usually no more than one year. Most short-term disability providers will require you to submit medical records to verify the disability claim. These can be requested through the doctor's office or the hospital's medical records department. Check with your loved one's employer's human resources department or your private disability insurance company to see if your loved one qualifies for short-term disability benefits.

Supplemental Security Income (SSI)

Stroke survivors who have contributed to Social Security through their paychecks may qualify for Supplemental Security Income (SSI) if their disability results in severe limitations that are expected to last longer than 12 months. SSI eligibility is based on income and financial resources (bank accounts, cash, real estate, etc.). If your loved one qualifies for SSI, they are eligible for your state's Medicaid program, which can help offset medical expenses.

Social Security Disability Insurance (SSDI)

Most stroke survivors qualify for Social Security benefits, such as Social Security Disability Insurance (SSDI), in addition to Supplemental Security Income (SSI). To be eligible for SSDI, your loved one must have been contributing to Social Security (typically deducted from their wages) and have passed a "recent work" test and "duration of work" test. Your loved one should apply for SSDI as soon as possible after their stroke because it can take up to five months for the Social Security Administration to process the application. Your loved one must be disabled for at least five full months before SSDI benefits can begin, and payment usually starts on the sixth month. The SSDI benefits will continue as long as your loved one's medical condition has not improved and they cannot work. However, these benefits may not continue indefinitely, as the Social Security Administration will review the case regularly to see if your loved one's disability continues to qualify. After your loved one receives SSDI for at least 24 months, they may be eligible for Medicare coverage.

Medication Assistance

The prohibitive cost of prescription medication can place a burden on any budget. Most stroke patients will go home taking several medications. Many pharmaceutical companies offer prescription assistance programs. Your loved one may qualify for a prescription drug card. If your loved one is receiving Medicare, they are already enrolled in Medicare Part D, which includes prescription drug coverage. You can't use a prescription discount card and Part D coverage at the same time. Use any prescription discount cards only when your loved one has reached their deductible limit or during a gap in coverage. Some states have state pharmaceutical assistance programs to help offset costs for eligible people. See the Medication Assistance resources section (page 160) for more information.

INSURANCE

Health insurance is essential for health promotion. Your loved one's health insurance will need to cover any hospital stays, rehabilitation services, and medication. In some instances, your loved one's health insurance may also need to cover post-acute care, such as long-term care in a nursing home.

Working with your loved one's case manager and social worker is key to getting the most from insurance coverage. All forms of insurance coverage are individualized to the medical necessity, and each health plan follows different criteria to provide services to its patients. Coverage for services may change depending on the patient's progress or medical necessity.

If you or your loved one feels that your insurance provider's decision is incorrect, you can file an appeal. Ask your insurance provider's case manager or social worker for directions on filing an appeal, or call member services and ask to speak to the appeals department.

Medicaid

Medicaid coverage is a state-based health insurance program that provides free or low-cost medical benefits. Medicaid programs may be called different things in each state. A stroke survivor may be eligible for coverage as a disabled person whose disability lasts for more than 12 months. If your loved one qualifies for Supplemental Security Income (SSI), they are eligible for Medicaid. Some states can grant presumptive eligibility to stroke survivors in the hospital if they are underinsured. Contact your state's Medicaid agency to apply for benefits.

Coverage varies from state to state and includes any combination of the following:

- Medical, dental, and vision coverage

- Some prescription drug coverage

- Inpatient rehabilitation

- Outpatient clinic rehabilitation

- Custodial and long-term care in a skilled nursing facility

- Durable medical equipment (DME)

- Select transportation services

Some states offer Medicaid programs for managed care organizations (MCOs). Enrollees receive health care through contracted in-network providers. There is no out-of-pocket payment for most covered services, but some plans may require co-pays. When your loved one first qualifies for Medicaid, they will be asked to select a health plan from a list. Plans may include enrollment in an MCO or fee-for-service coverage. Carefully review each plan with your loved one to determine what suits their needs.

Medicaid recipients may enroll in additional programs to support elder care or in-home support services. These programs often cover costs for services such as housecleaning, meal preparation, laundry, and shopping. Services may also include bathing, bowel and bladder care, and grooming. Coverage may even extend to include accompanying patients to medical appointments or protective supervision.

WHAT TO SAY ABOUT FINANCES

"Who do you think is the best person to help you with your finances?" Have an honest conversation with your loved one. Whom do they trust to help with finances? Distributing responsibility among other family members can ease responsibilities on the primary caregiver and help keep family members engaged in your loved one's care.

"Let's organize your bills and finances." Compile a list of your loved one's bills and bank accounts. Organize them in an easy-to-reference file or binder. Include account numbers and customer service numbers for all bills. Arrange for your loved one's financial designee to have the appropriate access to their accounts and bills.

"Let's review your beneficiaries." Remind your loved one that it may be time to update beneficiaries to their accounts. Create a plan with your loved one to review these regularly and update beneficiaries accordingly.

WHAT TO DO ABOUT FINANCES

Hold a family meeting. Family fights and tension about money issues are common. Conversations about money can be full of challenging emotions. When conflict about money is a possibility, holding a family meeting with an outside facilitator like a social worker or member of your faith community can help the family have a productive conversation.

Review finances and create a budget. Together with your loved one, review resources and create a budget for expenses. Are there family members who can contribute and help offset the costs of medical expenses?

Connect with the Patient Advocate Foundation (PAF). The healthcare system can be confusing, and you may have questions or need financial assistance. The PAF provides services for multiple medical conditions, including stroke. They have downloadable information and an online chat forum to ask questions and get answers, usually within the same day. See the Finances resources section (page 158) for more information.

Assistance for military veterans. If your loved one is a disabled veteran, contact the Department of Veterans Affairs to see what your loved one qualifies for.

Apply for everything. Put in an application for every financial assistance program you find, even if you don't think your loved one will qualify. You may be surprised what your loved one may be eligible for.

Monitor for financial abuse. Stroke survivors may be prone to elder fraud or financial exploitation. This may happen in the form of scammers or even individuals who were trusted to manage your loved one's finances. For tips on how to guard against financial abuse, visit the US Department of Justice's website. See the Finances resources section (page 158) for more information.

WHAT TO ASK THE FINANCIAL PLANNER

- Can you help us create a financial plan and budget?

- What resources can we qualify for?

- How can we offset medical expenses?

  If your loved one does not have a financial planner:

Discuss options with your loved one. Would they benefit from a financial planner, or is there someone they trust who can be a resource for questions?

Include all resources for funds in the budget and plan. Consider sources such as health insurance coverage, VA or military benefits, Social Security, workers' compensation, settlements, and investment accounts.

Medicare

Medicare is a government-sponsored insurance plan that covers people over the age of 65 or people who are disabled and receiving disability benefits for at least 24 months. Stroke survivors qualify for Medicare after 24 months of receiving Social Security Disability Insurance (SSDI). Medicare coverage is often divided into four parts:

1. **Medicare Part A** (inpatient care): This covers inpatient hospital stays, skilled nursing facilities with rehabilitation, skilled nursing services, laboratory tests, surgery, hospice, and home healthcare visits.

2. **Medicare Part B** (outpatient care): This covers outpatient care, home health care, preventive outpatient services, and durable medical equipment (DME).

3. **Medicare Advantage Plan** (formerly Medicare Part C): Patients enrolled in Medicare A and B may be enrolled in the Medicare Advantage Plan, run by a private insurance company that covers all of what traditional Medicare plans cover. The Medicare Advantage Plan may involve monthly fees. Some Medicare Advantage Plans may waive the 20 percent co-pay fees for healthcare services. Patients enrolled in this plan can only use designated healthcare providers in non-emergent situations, such as outpatient care.

4. **Medicare Part D** (prescription drug coverage): Patients enrolled in this plan may have a co-pay or minimum deductible each month. Prescription drugs can only be obtained at a designated pharmacy.

Since Medicare may only cover 80 percent of the cost for health care services, other secondary insurance providers may be added to help pay the 20 percent co-insurance fees. Insurance providers such as Medicaid, Medicare Supplemental Insurance (Medigap), or a private insurance carrier can help offset the remaining cost.

Commercial Insurance

Commercial insurance or private insurance carriers, such as Blue Cross Blue Shield, United Healthcare, or Humana, offer different health insurance packages. Coverage can be obtained through licensed agents, brokers, or your loved one's employer. Most health plans fall into two categories:

Health Maintenance Organization (HMO): These are managed healthcare plans covering services through a limited network of providers.

Preferred Provider Organization (PPO): These plans provide more flexibility in selecting providers. Staying within the contracted network of providers is usually lower in cost than an out-of-network provider.

LEGAL MATTERS

After a stroke is a good time for caregivers and stroke survivors to plan for the future if they have not done so already. The best scenario is when decisions are shared between a stroke survivor and loved ones as care partners. One day, your loved one may not be able to manage critical legal decisions about their care and will need to rely on someone to act in their best interests. Though the primary caregiver may be the natural choice to make these decisions, it may be best to hold a family meeting to discuss your loved one's decisions together. Plan ahead for critical decision-making and obtain the proper legal documents. This will make your loved one's wishes clear and prevent confusion later on.

Power of Attorney

A power of attorney (POA) is a document authorizing someone to make legal decisions for a loved one when they are no longer able. A POA can also grant authority to an individual to make financial decisions for a loved one.

Durable Power of Attorney for Health Care

This document goes into effect only when your loved one cannot make medical decisions for their own care. The designated person who holds durable power of attorney for health care can make all medical decisions for the loved one. This includes selecting medical treatment and healthcare providers, as well as making end-of-life decisions.

Advance Healthcare Directive or Living Will

An advance healthcare directive (AHCD), or living will, allows your loved one to state what kind of medical treatment they do and do not want to receive. This document can include what life support and resuscitation procedures your loved one would prefer not to have, such as tube feedings or ventilator support. In the event your loved one is admitted to a hospital or facility, they are often asked at the beginning of their stay if they have an advance directive or living will, which outlines healthcare wishes but does not include financial directives like a living trust.

AHCD forms are available at all hospitals and doctor's offices. Forms are specific to each state, and a free, state-specific AHCD can also be downloaded using an internet search. AHCDs do not need an attorney but must be signed by your loved one and witnessed by two people. In some states, an AHCD may need to be notarized. Creating a new AHCD replaces the previous one.

Living Trust

A living trust is a legal document that allows your loved one to create a trust and designate someone (a trustee) to manage the assets in the trust. A trust can be arranged in multiple ways and may specify how and when assets are passed to beneficiaries. Trusts can be set up so assets remain accessible to your loved one during their lifetime, with the remaining assets passed to beneficiaries after their death. With a living trust, beneficiaries may gain access to assets more quickly than using a will, since trusts usually avoid probate court proceedings.

WHAT TO SAY ABOUT INSURANCE

"We should look at your insurance coverage. Let's make sure you're getting the best care possible." Review your loved one's insurance plan regularly, especially during open enrollment periods.

WHAT TO DO ABOUT INSURANCE

Keep insurance coverage current. If there's a lapse in insurance coverage for more than two months, your loved one may be denied coverage for up to a year when signing up for a new plan or insurance carrier.

Apply for Medicaid right away. As with disability benefits, apply for Medicaid early. Ask the case manager at the hospital to help with this, or visit your state's Medicaid website to apply.

Shop around. If you are considering private insurance carriers or supplemental insurance, don't be afraid to shop around. Compare premium costs, co-pays, and deductibles against the type of coverage your loved one will need.

WHAT TO ASK THE INSURANCE PROVIDER'S CASE MANAGER

- Which case manager and social worker can we contact to help?

- What does our plan cover? Can you send us a summary?

- What are our co-pays? What are our deductibles?

- What kind of transportation services are covered?

- What other programs can we qualify for? Are there any programs specific to our state?

- What are our options for supplemental insurance coverage?

- Can you help us get in touch with county resources for seniors or disabled people?

Will

A will is a document that names an executor—a person who will manage your loved one's estate after their death. The executor of the will ensures the estate is settled according to your loved one's wishes. If your loved one does not have a will at the time of their death, state law will determine how property is distributed in probate court. This can include custody of minor children. Probate court proceedings can take six months to a year, depending on the state. Beneficiaries may not be granted anything until probate is complete.

Do Not Resuscitate (DNR)

A DNR is a doctor's order stating that you do not want to be resuscitated if you stop breathing or your heart stops beating. A discussion with your loved one's doctor is needed before such an order can be obtained. As a doctor's order, it must be followed, and paramedics and healthcare personnel are required to follow it. If your loved one does not have a DNR, healthcare personnel are required to do everything possible to resuscitate. DNR orders are usually completed in a hospital or long-term care facility, such as a nursing home or a skilled nursing facility.

Physician's Orders for Life-Sustaining Treatment (POLST)

A POLST is a doctor's order based on your loved one's wishes that tells healthcare personnel what to do in the event of an emergency. This document requires discussion with the doctor and can be changed and updated as your loved one's health status changes. POLST programs are run by each state and go by different names in each state. POLSTs are out-of-hospital medical orders that travel with your loved one wherever they go, such as home, the hospital, or skilled nursing facilities.

A POLST is different from an advance healthcare directive, because it is a doctor's order and does not require witnesses or notarization.

WHAT TO SAY ABOUT LEGAL MATTERS

"What medical treatments are acceptable to you?" Be open and honest and try to support your loved one's decisions the best way you can. These conversations may not be easy, so consulting with the doctor and trusted family members may help guide shared decision-making.

"Who is the best person to make healthcare decisions for you?" Talk to your loved one about who they trust to make medical decisions for them. If they are ever incapacitated, they need to feel confident about who will advocate for their care.

Things to say to ease conflict during conversations with family members or other key decision-makers:

"Thank you for taking the time to come." Showing appreciation when starting or restarting a discussion can begin things on a positive note.

"The goals of this discussion are . . ." Outline the goals at the beginning of the meeting. Why has the meeting been called? What are you trying to accomplish? Make sure that everyone agrees on the goals and redirect members to the core goal if the conversation goes off topic.

"What do you think are the best options?" Conflict can arise when someone doesn't feel like their input is being heard. Make sure to keep discussions inclusive of everyone involved.

"It sounds like we disagree. Why don't we spend five minutes coming up with different options? We can go over them and see which would work best." When in a disagreement, agree to disagree and refocus on how to move past it. Taking a team approach and coming up with solutions can help move the conversation forward without focusing on emotional conflict.

WHAT TO DO ABOUT LEGAL MATTERS

Consult an elder law attorney. An elder law attorney is recommended to help manage your loved one's legal matters and provide advice regarding legal documents. The National Elder Law Foundation (NELF) is a national organization that certifies elder care attorneys.

Hold a family meeting. Similar to meeting over finances, discussing legal matters also warrants a family meeting. Put in writing who will be responsible for which role—this will help keep the peace within the family and avoid bad communication.

Consider completing both a living trust and a will. A living trust covers assets and property outlined within the document. However, if your loved one acquires property before they die and does not include it in the trust, it will not pass under the trust document's terms. A will can include a clause that names a beneficiary to receive property not covered by the trust.

Organize important documents. Keep essential records in easy-to-access files, as well as other important documents, such as birth, death, or marriage certificates, divorce decrees, citizenship papers, property deeds, documents for funeral arrangements, military discharge papers, pension and retirement benefits, and medical and life insurance documents.

Keep original documents safe. Store your original documents in a fire- and water-resistant safe or box. Make sure this place is accessible to trusted family members.

WHAT TO ASK THE LAWYER

Questions to ask before hiring an elder law attorney:

- We would like to meet with you for an initial consultation. What are your fees?

- What kind of legal services do you provide? (For example, estate planning, long-term care planning, help in the event of elder abuse or financial elder abuse, etc.)

- What credentials do you hold? (For example, Certified Elder Law Attorney, or CELA)

- How long have you been in practice, and where?

- Are you a member of any relevant organizations? (For instance, National Academy of Elder Law Attorneys)

- If a legal document needs to be defended in court, will you litigate it?

- How familiar are you with Medicare and Medicaid laws?

- What type of training does your firm have for paralegals assigned to our case?

- Do you make home visits?

Questions to ask your elder law attorney:

- What are the requirements for mental capacity before my loved one can sign legal documents?

- How much preparation is needed on our part?

- How do we protect our assets?

- What kind of financial protections can we have from creditors?

- How do we avoid estate taxes?

- Can you go over the probate process so we can better understand it?

- Can you help with probate?

- How can we reach you if we need help? Who is our main point of contact?

HOW ARE YOU DOING?

This chapter went over some serious subject matter that can be emotionally draining. Discussions over financial and legal decision-making can stir up feelings that are hard to process. Conflict may arise as family members express their views, and emotions often run high. If family meetings become unproductive, consider involving a social worker or a member of your faith community to help guide the discussion. As difficult as it is to have these conversations, they must be had, ideally before your loved one becomes too incapacitated to make decisions. Planning ahead and making sure that your loved one is part of the shared decision-making can prevent confusion and conflict. It's better to make sure everyone is on the same page instead of arguing after your loved one cannot make their wishes known.

You may feel conflicted about some of the care decisions your loved one wants. As their care partner, you can voice your concerns in an open and honest dialogue. Make your views known, and do your best to support your loved one's final decision.

Take a moment to pause and allow yourself a few minutes of peace and quiet. Studies show that pausing for even just 20 minutes a day can decrease stress symptoms by almost half. It does not have to be 20 consecutive minutes, but a total of 20 minutes a day. Try spending five minutes slowly relaxing your muscles while sitting in your car listening to music, or five minutes of breathing exercises while waiting in line. Other activities that can help are saying a prayer, playing with a pet, or singing a song. Whatever combination of activities you do to pause and relax can count toward your 20 minutes.

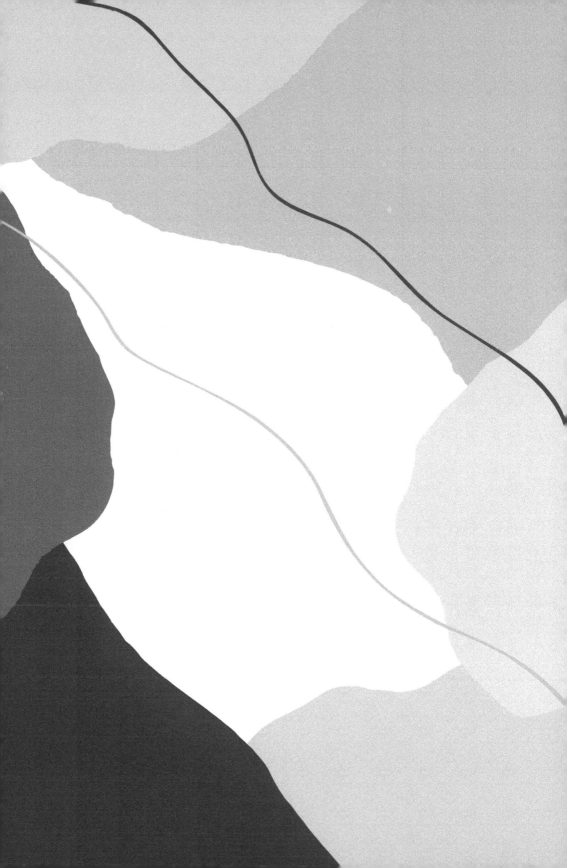

CHAPTER 8

LONG-TERM CAREGIVING HELP

Stefan

I f you follow me, I'll show you the cafeteria," the tour guide directed. Stefan nodded and silently trailed after her. This was the third nursing home he'd visited today, and this tour guide seemed just like all the rest. He couldn't remember her name, though she seemed nice enough.

He glanced at the generic wall art mounted on the cream-colored walls. He thought he saw the same pictures at the first nursing home he visited. He drew a deep breath and tried to pay attention to what his tour guide was saying, but he didn't have much hope for this nursing home, either. He couldn't imagine placing Nana here.

Stefan's grandmother, his nana, had a stroke four years earlier that left her bedridden and unable to communicate. Nana lived with him and his wife, Gillian, and Gillian was primarily responsible for Nana's day-to-day care. A week ago, Gillian tore her rotator cuff while repositioning Nana in bed and needed surgery. With his full-time job and his wife's injury, neither he nor Gillian could continue caring for Nana. So today he was touring nursing homes as possible places for Nana to get the care she needed.

"Here's the cafeteria," the tour guide told him. Stefan walked around the room, inspecting the area while the tour guide talked about the meals offered here. There was nothing wrong with any of the nursing homes he visited so far, but Stefan was hesitant to send Nana to any of them. He wondered how much of what he was feeling was because of his long-time reluctance to place Nana in a nursing home.

"Do you have any questions for me?" his tour guide asked.

"No, I don't," Stefan said. "Thank you so much for your time."

"Feel free to contact me if you have any questions."

"Great," said Stefan. "I will."

Later in the car, Stefan stretched his neck from side to side and took a deep breath. He hoped to find a place he felt comfortable with soon.

"Two more nursing homes to go," he told himself, then started his car.

GETTING ADDITIONAL CAREGIVING HELP

Regardless of what kind of care you provide to your loved one, getting outside caregiving help, whether from family or an agency, can help you maintain a work-life balance and free you up for other activities. You don't have to do everything yourself. Use the resources around you as much as you can.

When you need breaks from caregiving, your insurance provider may be able to cover adult day services or respite care services for your loved one. Adult day service centers provide health monitoring and assistance with daily activities while providing activities and socialization for your loved one. Respite care provides a temporary break for caregivers. Such care for your loved one can be provided at home, at an adult day center, or in a healthcare facility, and can be arranged for a day or a few weeks.

Getting help with transportation services can relieve some of the caregiver strain. Ask your insurance provider if transportation services can take your loved one to medical appointments and services or be used for general transportation purposes. Some public transit services offer pickups for people with disabilities.

The US Administration on Aging's Eldercare Locator can help find resources in your community on their website—see the Government Assistance resources on page 159. The Eldercare Locator can help you find resources such as transportation services, meal preparation services, and caregiver support programs. Consider other services to help with household management, such as grocery delivery, housekeeping, or lawn care.

WHAT TO SAY TO YOUR LOVED ONE ABOUT GETTING OUTSIDE HELP

"Help me understand your concerns." Listen to your loved one's concerns and address them. Some stroke survivors may be reluctant to accept help from strangers or they don't want strangers in their home. Reassure your loved one that you need help and that hiring someone does not mean that you will abandon them.

"It will make me feel better if there is someone who can help you during part of the day." If your loved one lives alone and is unwilling to accept help, reassure them that this is something they can do to help you care for them.

"How about we try a housekeeper for a week and see how it goes?" Sometimes it's easier for your loved one to accept help with housework before they are willing to have someone help with personal care. Taking things step by step with trial periods will help your loved one become familiar with their attendant and build trust.

WHAT TO DO WHEN SEEKING HELP

When seeking additional caregiving help, consider your needs as a caregiver as well as the needs of your loved one. Assess these areas of need to see where you may need help:

Personal care: activities of daily living, such as eating, dressing, toileting, bathing, and grooming

Health care: assistance with rehabilitation therapy, medical appointments, transportation, and medication management

Household management: household finances, cleaning, laundry, cooking, shopping, lawn care, pet care

Emotional support: companionship and socialization, conversation, meaningful activities, hobbies

WHAT TO ASK A POTENTIAL SERVICE PROVIDER

- What services are you willing to provide?

- Where have you worked before?

- What are your credentials? What kind of training have you received?

- Can you provide me with two work-related references and one personal reference I can contact?

- Do you have a car? Can you show me proof of insurance and a driver's license?

- How do you handle someone who is stubborn, angry, or fearful?

LONG-TERM CARE

For some stroke survivors and their families, there may be a need for long-term care. A stroke survivor and caregiver must carefully weigh the options and determine the best fit. Some stroke survivors may also feel hesitant to use long-term-care providers due to a desire to retain as much independence as they can. In any decision regarding long-term care, the decision should be shared among your loved one, caregivers, and family.

One option for long-term care is to hire paid in-home caregivers, known as "personal care assistants" or "home health aides." These aides can assist your loved one with personal care, such as bathing, toileting, and grooming. They may perform household management tasks, such as grocery shopping, meal preparation, and light housekeeping. Some programs that provide in-home support services, such as part-time caregivers, are covered by insurance. However, if your loved one requires more help from a personal care aide, the cost is usually out of pocket and varies depending on how much help is needed. The Family

Caregiver Alliance has a great guide on hiring in-home help on their website—see the Caregivers resources on page 157.

Stroke survivors who can no longer live alone but don't need daily medical care may benefit from an assisted living facility. Assisted living facilities can offer healthcare services, such as rehabilitation therapy from physical, occupational, and speech therapists; mental health services; and a pharmacy. Staff can assist with laundry, meals, housekeeping, and transportation. Often, an assisted living facility offers programs on wellness and exercise, planned outings, and social activities. In some states, Medicaid can offer financial aid for low-income residents. The cost for an assisted living facility is not usually covered by Medicare.

Nursing homes, or skilled nursing facilities (SNFs), offer care to people who require full-time medical care and monitoring. SNFs provide help with meals, bathing, grooming, dressing, and 24/7 medical supervision. Medicare will cover short-term stays at an SNF for rehabilitation but may not cover long-term residency. In most cases, Medicaid covers long-term care at an SNF.

WHAT TO SAY ABOUT LONG TERM CARE

"I know this is difficult. We need to decide on the best way to keep you safe." Focusing the conversation on the best scenario to keep them safe may help ease your loved one's fears.

"How do you feel about this? What are your thoughts or concerns?" Letting your loved one voice their thoughts or concerns can make them feel heard and help you understand how they are feeling.

HOW TO CHOOSE A CARE FACILITY

Tour facilities with your loved one, if possible. Visit the facility multiple times, at different times of the day, if possible, to get a clearer view of the care provided.

Check for cleanliness. Check the bathrooms, both the ones for general use and in the resident rooms.

Talk to residents and visiting family members at the facilities. Residents and family members may give you more insight into what goes on in the facility.

Pay attention to staff interactions. How staff interacts with the residents is important. Do they treat them with kindness and respect?

Check the activities calendar. Are all the activities in-house, or do they provide outings for a change in scenery?

Visit the cafeteria. What kind of meals do they serve? Do they allow meals from home?

WHAT TO ASK
A LONG-TERM CARE PROVIDER

- What credentials does the staff have? What kind of training is required?

- What experience does your staff have working with stroke survivors?

- What kind of services does your facility provide?

- What activities and programs can residents participate in?

- Do you provide transportation services?

- What kind of rehabilitation services does your facility offer?

- What insurance providers do you accept?

- Are there any financial aid programs we could qualify for?

- Can you describe a typical day for my loved one?

- How will I be kept informed of my loved one's condition?

- What personal belongings can my loved one bring?

- Can you tell me about the visitation policy?

HOW ARE YOU DOING?

As a caregiver, knowing your limits is an essential part of caregiving. Be honest about what you can and can't do—this benefits yourself and your loved one. Don't be afraid to seek help from friends, family, or paid services. Guilt over taking some time for yourself has no place here— you can't help your loved one if you are not at your best in mind, body, and spirit.

When you find some free time, you may be at a loss as to how to spend it or where to even start. Create a list of activities to help guide your decision. Start with the following categories: 15 minutes, 30 minutes, 45 minutes, 1 hour, 2 hours, half a day, and one day. Brainstorm and write down things that you can do just for yourself in those time frames. For example, in 15 minutes you can meditate, take a warm shower, play a game on your phone, or call a friend for a quick chat. When you have 30 minutes to yourself, you may be able to take a walk, read a magazine or a few chapters of a good book, or watch an episode of your favorite show. Fill this list with things you enjoy doing. Once you are done, you have a ready-made guide, reminding you of things you can do for your own enjoyment whenever the opportunity arises. Spend time treating yourself in small moments during the day or pampering yourself with a day of planned activities.

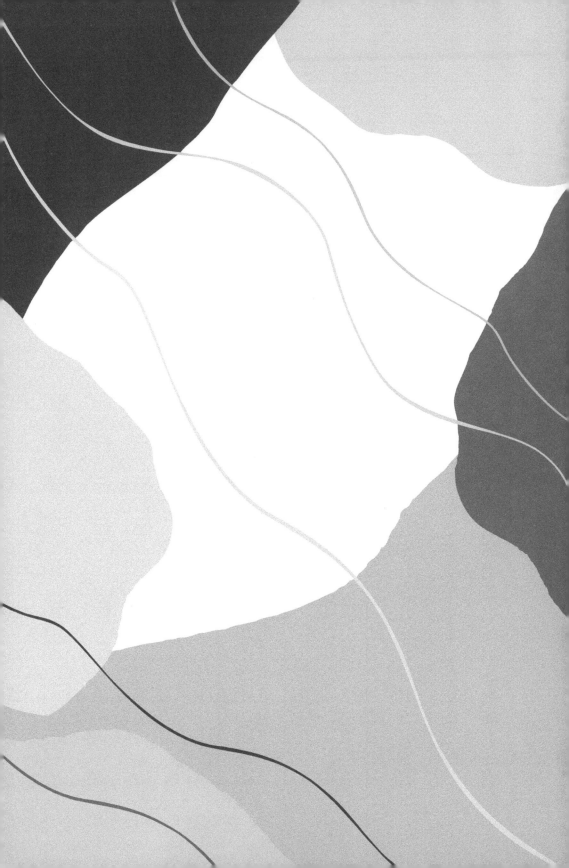

PART THREE

CARING FOR YOURSELF

CHAPTER 9

HOW CAREGIVING AFFECTS YOU

Rosalyn

Rosalyn flopped wearily on her bed. She lay on her back, arms and legs spread wide, unmoving. She stared at the ceiling, not blinking. She was too tired to blink. Every muscle ached, and her heart sat heavy in her chest. Silent tears pooled in her eyes and began to stream from the corners of her eyes. The tears spilled downward and wet her hair. She didn't care.

Rosalyn has been the primary caregiver for her elderly mother, Lorraine, for the last three years. Lorraine suffered a major stroke, which left her unable to move the right side of her body. Rosalyn did everything for her mom. Turning, feeding, cleaning up after her mom, you name it. She managed Lorraine's meager Social Security check and used it to offset the cost of her mom's medications. Anything Lorraine needed, Rosalyn did. It's what she had always done.

But she was exhausted. Rosalyn's brother and sister hardly came over to help. She was a housewife, they said, and should be able to take care of Mom because she was home all day anyway. As a result, she was constantly in motion, between taking care of Lorraine and managing her kids' busy schedules and homework. Rosalyn hardly saw her husband anymore, since he worked two jobs so she could stay home to take care of Lorraine and the kids.

The bedroom door opened softly. "Ros?" her husband, Peter, whispered. "Why are you still up? Are you okay?"

Rosalyn's eyes slowly met Peter's. He was home? How long had she been lying here staring at the ceiling? Peter looked at her tear-streaked face with concern.

"You need a break," he said. "I think it's time we look into respite care."

THE PHYSICAL AND EMOTIONAL TOLL

A caregiver's quality of life is dependent on maintaining a balance among physical, mental, emotional, and spiritual well-being.

Caregiver tasks are many, and often, a caregiver does "whatever needs to be done." Depending on your loved one's needs, caregiver duties could include any combination of the following:

Activities of daily living: assisting with feeding, dressing, grooming, bathing, toileting, medication management, mobility and transfers, and helping with exercises for stroke recovery

Household management: food preparation, housekeeping, laundry, shopping, and transportation

Financial, legal, and medical care: managing finances and accounts, meeting with financial planners or advisors, arranging for appropriate legal documents, and coordinating medical appointments

Research: exploring available care services or disease information

Emotional, social, and spiritual support: being a care companion and providing emotional support, arranging for socialization and spiritual support for your loved one

Caregiving can be a challenging and tiring job, often resulting in constant stress on your body. A caregiver has to be vigilant not to hurt themself or push their body too far. Fatigue, caregiver burnout, and sleep problems can develop when caregivers don't actively take the time to care for themselves. Physical symptoms, such as tension, headaches, and tight muscles in the shoulders or neck, can emerge.

When a caregiver has complicated interactions with the people around them, it can impact their mental well-being. Dealing with a confused loved one or a family member who is in denial about your loved one's condition can be difficult. Tension with family members over financial issues or care decisions can weigh heavily on a caregiver's mind.

Caregivers can experience a wide range of emotions, including guilt, anger, frustration, resentment, and depression. These emotions are complex, challenging, and, above all, completely normal. You shouldn't feel bad about feeling this way. When emotions become difficult to deal with, reach out to family and friends and let them know how you feel and what you are going through. Sometimes it's difficult to identify what you are feeling, and you may not recognize your feelings or understand them yourself. Talking to someone and unburdening yourself of the emotional strain can help. In some cases, seeking professional guidance or speaking with a religious advisor can be very helpful.

Caregivers who aren't meeting their spiritual needs can feel isolated and uncertain. When a caregiver doesn't make time to connect with their religious advisors or members of their faith, they can lose a significant part of their support system. Prayer or meditation can be a great comfort and balm to a weary heart when you are feeling alone.

Taking care of yourself should be a high priority. In the care partnership, you are not just taking care of your loved one; you are also taking care of yourself. You and your loved one are figuring out how to be your best selves in a new stage in life. Be kind to yourself and treat yourself as you would a good friend. You deserve it.

Stress and Anxiety

Worrying is normal, but it can be hard to focus or even function when worries become difficult to push away and troubling thoughts take over. Anxiety and feelings of helplessness can make it challenging to think or act. Sometimes, you can experience physical symptoms, such as tense muscles, tremors, or heart palpitations. Anxiety can make it difficult to sleep at night and leave you tired and inattentive during the day.

One of the best treatments for anxiety is exercise. Exercise releases endorphins in our bloodstream that boost our mood and help calm the mind. Brisk exercise such as walking, swimming, or a fitness class can be a great way to elevate your spirits and improve overall physical health. Relaxation techniques like meditation and breathing exercises can also help calm the mind. Yoga has the dual benefit of exercise and mindfulness.

If your anxiety gets too overwhelming, visit your primary care physician and request an evaluation. Your doctor may be able to recommend cognitive and behavioral treatments or prescribe medications to help with anxiety.

Frustration and Anger

Some days it's just plain hard. Your loved one is being particularly stubborn about taking their medication, or you keep getting the runaround when you call the doctor's office. There are days when you are upset because your role is not recognized, and you feel helpless or isolated. It's easy and normal to feel frustrated in any given situation. But when frustrations continue to build, it can lead to anger.

The first thing is to acknowledge that anger is an entirely normal reaction. When fatigue sets in from the daily grind and the emotional toll, it can leave you emotionally exhausted. When this happens, it becomes more challenging to hold your temper and remain calm. Anger is a complex emotion, and it's natural to feel angry at some point in your caregiver journey. Don't feel guilty or punish yourself when you feel this way. Remember the countless times you were considerate and patient. Allow yourself these moments of imperfection—we all have them.

When you are feeling angry, you need a healthy way to release your anger. Writing down your feelings or going into another room to let out what you want to say can help. Find an outlet that works for you, some form of release that can lift your mood. Try not to spend time brooding over things that you have no control over. Instead, focus on something you can control: that is, your reaction and attitude about the situation. How you deal with a problem depends mainly on your interpretation and your response.

Sadness and Depression

When the physical and emotional toll becomes too much, caregivers can experience negative emotions that can lead to depression. Unfortunately, feelings of sadness and depression are often downplayed. People may tell you to "get over it" or "it's all in your head" instead of seeing sadness or depression as a sign that something is wrong. Ignoring feelings of sadness and depression does not make them go away. Denial of those feelings only perpetuates the myth that mental health issues are not real or valid. Depression is very real, and an estimated 20 percent of caregivers suffer from depression.

Symptoms of depression may include:

- A change in eating habits that results in weight gain or weight loss

- Feeling tired and sleeping too much or too little

- Feeling that nothing you do is good enough

- Diminished interest In people or activities

If these symptoms persist for more than two weeks, it is best to see a doctor and get treatment.

While undergoing treatment, you will likely need some time to see improvement. Let friends and family help you. Find someone to confide in to help relieve your burden. Feeling better doesn't happen overnight, but with treatment, self-care, and support, you can expect to feel a little bit better each day.

Guilt

Some caregivers have a self-imposed sense of duty to their loved one. They feel that caregiving is their personal responsibility because no one else can do it or because there is no room in their finances to hire a professional caregiver. Most caregivers have difficulty saying no to the job. In some cases, caregivers feel pressured to perform caregiving tasks by their loved one or another family member. Caregivers may feel guilty for having negative emotions, such as anger or resentment.

It's normal to feel guilty sometimes—many caregivers do. Start by acknowledging the guilt to move forward. Forgive yourself for being an imperfect person. You are doing your best, and that is what matters. Wallowing in your guilt helps no one and slowly eats away at your soul. You are good enough.

Exhaustion and Physical Issues

Caregiver burnout can be a tipping point for caregivers. When a caregiver's physical, mental, social, and spiritual needs are not being met, the overwhelming stress can lead to feelings of helplessness and exhaustion. When a caregiver is focused on their loved one's care, sometimes they don't realize that their own health and well-being are suffering. Caregiver burnout combines all the feelings already mentioned—anxiety, anger, frustration, depression, and guilt—leaving the caregiver feeling wrung out and utterly exhausted.

Caregivers can experience any combination of the following signs of exhaustion and burnout:

- Feeling overwhelmed

- Constantly worrying

- Feeling tired or exhausted often

- Losing sleep or sleeping too much

- Unplanned weight gain or weight loss

- Becoming short-tempered or easily irritated

- Losing interest in things you used to enjoy

- Feeling depressed or sad

- Frequent headaches or body pain

- Alcohol abuse

- Drug abuse (including prescription drugs)

If you feel overwhelmed and exhausted, it's time to take a break—a real one. It may be challenging to picture leaving your loved one under someone else's care, but you need relief. Arrange for respite care at a facility or a short stay at a nursing home and take a break for a few days.

As your caregiver journey continues, these feelings may return from time to time. It is essential to establish healthy routines, be on the lookout for signs of caregiver burnout, and seek help when you need it.

WHAT TO DO ABOUT CAREGIVER BURNOUT

Take care of yourself. Set personal health goals for yourself. Goals can include finding time to exercise a few days a week, eating a healthier diet, drinking more water, or establishing a healthy sleep routine.

Enlist others. Permit yourself to ask for and accept help from others. Sometimes it's hard to let go of duties that we think only we can handle. Make a list of things people can help you with, and let them choose what they can handle.

Give yourself a break. Don't just give yourself a physical break; give yourself a break from negative thoughts as well. Don't be so hard on yourself. You are doing the best you can and making the best decisions possible for you and your loved one.

Create a support system. Develop a core group of people you trust. Stay connected with people who can be a source of support and encouragement. Join a stroke or caregiver support group or seek comfort and advice from your local religious organization.

Set realistic goals. Divide large tasks into smaller steps. Complex tasks don't seem so bad when you can feel good about making progress toward completing them.

Learn to say no. It's okay to set limits and tell people no when a request is too draining on you. Focus on what you can realistically do. By saying no, you are setting boundaries and giving yourself a gift.

Say yes when someone offers help. Don't be shy about accepting help. Anything that reduces your responsibilities or makes tasks easier is also a gift and will reduce caregiver strain.

WHAT TO ASK THE DOCTOR OR NURSE

- Are there any resources that can help me reduce caregiver strain?

- What are some things I should do to avoid caregiver burnout?

GRIEF AND LOSS

Most people associate grief and loss with death. However, feelings of grief and loss can develop even when your loved one is very much alive. When a loved one suffers from a stroke, their physical and mental abilities change. For some caregivers, this can be difficult to watch. Seeing your loved one change and become less of their former self can stir feelings of loss.

Caregivers can also feel a sense of loss within their own life—a loss of independence or control. When taking on a caregiver role, a sense of grief and loss over your former self and future plans can develop. Ignoring feelings of loss can lead to sadness and despair or anger and resentment.

When our loved ones die, grief can be intense. There is no fixed length of time that a person needs to grieve. Everyone grieves differently. Some cultures and faiths have different rituals for the grieving process. Many caregivers seek solace from their family, friends, or faith community. There is no "correct" way to mourn, since the grieving process is an intensely personal experience. It's important to take as much time as you need and not listen to anyone who tells you how to grieve or when is enough.

Symptoms of grief can manifest in different ways. Crying, poor appetite, and sleeplessness are common symptoms. Feelings of emptiness or heaviness can leave the grieving individual feeling weak and weary. Some may feel alone or angry that others are moving on while their life seems at a standstill. Others may wish to separate themselves from their grief and push themselves into increased activity so they can't think about their feelings.

WHAT TO DO ABOUT GRIEF

Write it down. Expressing yourself through writing can help deal with complex feelings, especially if you combine it with a gratitude journal and remember things you are thankful for.

Talk to someone. Speaking with a trusted friend or advisor can help process these feelings and begin to heal.

Establish a routine. A routine of meditation, exercise, or prayer can help calm intense feelings of grief.

HOW ARE YOU DOING?

Some days are easy, and other days are challenging. No, I'm not referring to caregiving—I'm talking about taking the time to take care of yourself. It can be difficult to turn the lens on yourself and really examine how you are doing. Sometimes it can be hard to allow yourself this time. Give yourself permission to take care of yourself.

I've talked about writing thoughts down to help you process emotions, but sometimes even that can be difficult for some people. Consider recording your thoughts and talking them out, either on an audio recorder or on video. Journaling doesn't have to mean putting your thoughts on paper. The whole point of journaling is to release your thoughts. Sometimes just speaking them out loud is therapeutic. It allows you to acknowledge the existence of complex feelings and gives a name to them. Once you recognize your emotions, you can begin dealing with them.

CHAPTER 10

WORK-LIFE BALANCE

Jasmine

G randpa's medication schedule is on the counter," Jasmine said as she put the last few water bottles in the small ice chest. She added an extra ice pack as an afterthought.

"Yes, Auntie," sighed Haley. "I saw it the first time you pointed it out."

Jasmine closed the lid on the ice chest and heaved it off the kitchen counter. Maybe she should add another sandwich? Haley grabbed the handle of the ice chest and grunted as she pulled it away.

"Geez, Auntie Jasmine. What did you pack? This thing is a lot heavier than it looks." Jasmine didn't hear her. She was too busy double-checking the contents of her giant tote bag.

"Don't forget to check Grandpa's blood sugar before lunch and log it in the book," Jasmine continued. "Grandpa's lunch is in the microwave. Just heat it up. I left you sandwiches in the fridge. His physical therapist should be coming this afternoon. Extra movies are on the coffee table. Remind him to use his walker, even if he doesn't want to. He'll insist he doesn't need it. He does. He can have the crackers and cheese in the container in the fridge if he wants a snack. Oh! His favorite tea is in the pantry on the second shelf. Don't let him put sugar in his tea. He's diabetic. Don't forget his medication schedule—"

Jasmine stopped abruptly as Haley's hands closed over her own. She looked up, staring into her niece's eyes.

"Is on the kitchen counter," Haley finished Jasmine's sentence. Haley ushered Jasmine out the door and helped her put the ice chest and tote bag in the car next to the beach chair and picnic blanket.

"Honestly, Auntie Jasmine, it's going to be fine. You're only going to be gone half a day. It's not like I haven't helped take care of Grandpa before. Now get out of here before you change your mind."

Jasmine obediently climbed in the car. This was the first time she had more than 30 minutes to herself in months. She was planning to relax at the beach for a few hours. Sand, surf, and a good book. Still, she couldn't help but feel a little guilty, but she reminded herself that she needed to take care of herself, too. Haley can handle it, she told herself. Taking a deep breath, Jasmine turned the key in the ignition.

"This is for me," she said. Her dad's face flashed momentarily in her mind. "This is for *us*," she amended, and pulled the car out of the driveway.

BALANCING WORK AND CAREGIVING

Balancing work and life is pretty hard already. When you add care-giving to the mix, it may seem like more than you can handle. You're not alone. It is estimated that 60 percent of caregivers of adults 50 or older also have a full- or part-time job. Regardless of what level of care you provide to your loved one, you need a game plan to manage caregiving and work.

Getting organized should be a top priority. You have a lot on your to-do list, so a system to keep track of everything is essential. A family calendar is a good way to keep everyone informed about what's happening. There are many apps available for shared calendars.

It is important to inform your manager and co-workers of your caregiving responsibilities. Explaining that you are a caregiver for your loved one and what duties you may have can make your workplace aware and understanding of your situation. Read the employee handbook and get to know your company rules regarding time off and leave requests. The company may also have policies or programs for care-givers that allow family leave requests or flexible work options.

The Family and Medical Leave Act (FMLA) can allow you to take time off to care for your loved one. FMLA enables you to take up to 12 weeks off work every year without pay and still retain your job. If your employer is covered under FMLA, they are required to keep up your health insurance coverage while you are out on FMLA leave. However, you may still need to pay your portion of the health insurance premiums.

HOW TO BALANCE WORK AND CAREGIVING

Have a conversation with your boss. Schedule a meeting to speak to them about your caregiver responsibilities. Let them know that you are the caregiver for your loved one but that you continue to take your commitment to the workplace seriously. Make sure your boss knows you have a plan for getting your work done.

Keep work and home separate. As much as possible, perform caregiving tasks on personal time instead of work hours. Schedule calls on your break time or on lunch, and try to keep appointments limited to your days off.

WHAT TO ASK YOUR MANAGER OR HR DEPARTMENT

- Are there options for flexible work schedules?

- What are our policies regarding FMLA?

- Who is considered "immediate family" under FMLA?

Your employer is not required to pay you during FMLA leave, so you may choose to use your paid time off to cover expenses. Depending on company policy, your employer may require you to use your vacation time first. To learn more about FMLA, see the Caregivers resources section (page 157).

ASKING FOR HELP

Asking for help is difficult for some caregivers. Some caregivers may feel that they need to do everything themselves or are the only ones who can provide the best care. They may not know what kind of help to ask for or feel guilty asking for help. But it's not about doing everything yourself. As a caregiver, you are the ultimate *coordinator* of your loved one's care. To do that effectively requires the ability to ask for help and delegate tasks appropriately.

As a caregiver, you may have the tendency to put others ahead of your own needs. It is best to ask for help before you feel exhausted, overwhelmed, or helpless. There is an entire community of people around you who can help.

When asking for help, try not to ask at the last minute. Give your friends and family advance notice so they can adjust their schedule. Explain why you need help. People are usually happy to help if they understand the situation. Remember to ask for what you know that person can give.

Some helpers will be more confident performing their tasks than others. Give clear instructions. This could be as simple as a grocery list for someone going to the store for you. Or it can be a complete set of instructions for preparing a meal or giving medications. When asking someone to perform a more complex task, have everything they need prepared for them, like organizing medications on a tray. Providing a menu with details for snacks and meals can give your helper confidence and make them more likely to help you again. If your helper assists with transportation to a doctor's appointment, offer written instructions about the appointment and include any advice on details like helping your loved one in and out of the car. When possible, walk a helper through some of the more complex tasks to ensure that things go smoothly.

AVAILABLE OUTSIDE SERVICES

While your friends and family may be your first line of people to ask for help, other options are available within your community. Community resources can help lighten the non-caregiving load, such as housekeeping, meal preparation, lawn care, or shopping. An internet search will bring up information regarding services near you. Consider joining a social media group in your area and requesting referrals for services

HOW TO ASK FOR HELP

Divide and conquer. Create a list of things that need to be done. Divide the tasks among everyone willing to help.

Establish a shared to-do list. There are many apps available that can organize tasks. Some apps allow you to create a to-do list that can be shared with others.

WHAT TO ASK YOUR FAMILY AND FRIENDS

- Can you go to the grocery store/pharmacy for me?

- What would you like to do to help?

- Do you know how grateful I am? I couldn't have done this without you.

you need. This can provide valuable connections with other local residents who can share their experiences.

Housekeeping and gardening services can help you maintain your household and free up time. Cleaning services can be personalized to fit your budget and range from once a week to monthly services. The kitchen and bathrooms tend to be the most labor-intensive to clean, so even having someone clean them once a month can be a huge relief.

The time you spend cooking can be reduced by enlisting meal preparation services. Meals on Wheels is a popular meal delivery service that provides pre-packaged, fully cooked meals that may be covered by Medicare for eligible adults. Payment plans are available for individuals who don't meet Medicare coverage requirements. If your budget allows, meal-kit delivery services can be a time-saver. These services deliver pre-packaged ingredients and cooking instructions for each meal.

Time spent grocery shopping can also be reduced. Most grocery stores offer curbside pickup at the store or delivery services if you order through their website. The fee for this service is usually offset by the fact that you save money that would otherwise be spent on impulse purchases at the store.

HOW ARE YOU DOING?

Caregivers seem to have a certain sense of duty and selflessness in their psyche that makes it difficult for them to accept help. Rest assured, you don't have to do everything by yourself, and you are most definitely worthy of receiving help.

WHAT TO DO TO HIRE HELP

Assess your needs. What do you need help with? Yes, you can do it yourself, but how much stress and time will it relieve by employing these services?

Comparison-shop. Do your research for each prospective service provider. Will they fit your needs? Are they within your budget? Is there a promo code available?

WHAT TO ASK
PROSPECTIVE SERVICE PROVIDERS

- What kind of services do you provide?

- What is the cost?

- How do you prefer to be paid?

- How long have you been in business?

- How large is your staff?

- Do you have any references we can contact?

- Can you provide examples of your previous work?

Developing your relationships with your friends and family can make it easier to ask for help. Reaching out to your community becomes easier as you make new friends and connections. Socializing is a basic human need. By creating bonds within your community, you can fulfill the social needs of both you and your loved one. Your support community can be a vital resource for obtaining specific help, asking questions, or just getting encouragement and support from others who can relate. Social media platforms have many relevant social groups you can join. Don't limit yourself to stroke- or caregiver-related groups, but also look into groups related to any hobbies you may have. You are more than a caregiver—you're a unique individual with varied interests who can share in connections with other like-minded people.

One last suggestion: Make an effort to schedule a get-together with friends and family at least once a month. This can be a family dinner, a book club meeting, or an impromptu meetup for a cup of coffee. The important thing is to leave the house for a change of scenery and connect with people whose company you enjoy.

CHAPTER 11

STAYING HEALTHY AND RESILIENT

Selma

Selma fidgeted nervously in her chair. This was her first stroke support group meeting, and it was almost her turn. She didn't know what to say.

"Selma," Gaby, the social worker, called on her. "Can you tell us what brings you here today?" Six pairs of eyes fixed on Selma.

"I'm not really sure why I'm here," Selma swallowed hard. "My mom had her stroke a year ago. I take care of her because everyone else in the family lives far away. My mom's doctor said it would be a good thing for me to come, so here I am."

"What is an average day like for you?" the woman sitting next to her asked.

"I help my mom with everything," Selma started. "She can't move the right side of her body. I change her diapers, take her to the bathroom, get her dressed, make her food, and help her eat. I also help her with physical therapy, give her meds, and take her to her doctor appointments. In the evening, I help the kids with homework and give my mom a bath before I go to bed myself."

"Sounds like a lot," the woman murmured. "When was the last time you did something for yourself?"

Selma blinked. *When was the last time?* she thought. "I don't remember."

The woman gave her an understanding smile. "It sounds like you haven't taken any time to care for yourself. Are you tired all the time?"

Selma nodded. She didn't realize how exhausted she was until the woman asked her.

The woman reached out and gently took her hand. "You can't be a good caregiver if you don't take care of yourself first. That's a lesson we've all had to learn."

"I'm so tired all the time. I don't really have any energy or desire to do more," Selma said.

"Let us give you some advice—we've been there and we're all here to help."

GET MOVING

Regular exercise will reduce your stress levels and keep you healthy and fit. Do anything that moves you! Jump up and go for a brisk walk or follow a workout video. By moving your body, even just for 20 minutes, at least three times a week, you'll get your body moving, strengthen your heart, and improve your stamina.

Take every opportunity to move your body. Dance while you vacuum or sweep the patio, stretch or do a few squats during a commercial, or use a treadmill or stationary bike while watching TV. Jog to the mailbox and back every day instead of walking. Set aside 10 minutes a day to stretch. Get moving, even while doing small tasks around the house. Every bit counts.

Yoga and tai chi are beneficial to both stroke survivors and caregivers, so this is something you can do together with your loved one. Check out videos on the internet for yoga and tai chi for stroke recovery.

WHAT TO DO TO GET EXERCISE

- **Make it social.** Join community-based groups or apps that allow you to share progress—this can keep you motivated. Some include Facebook, MyFitnessPal, Fitbit, and Yes.Fit.

- **Get creative.** Some options include:

  - **Go on a virtual run.** Join a virtual run community and complete virtual runs to earn actual marathon medals. Virtual marathons can be completed at your own pace. Virtual marathons can be as short as 1K and fees can start as low as $10. To sign up, search the internet or the app store on your smartphone for "virtual run."

  - **Add geocaching to your hike.** Geocaching is a global activity that involves finding hidden places using a GPS. Check out Geocaching.com to learn more.

  - **Kayak, canoe, or raft.** If you love being on the water, you don't need to spend thousands of dollars. Consider investing in a small kayak and a life jacket. Boating can be great exercise and a transformative escape from the pressures of life.

  - **Go hiking.** Exercise while enjoying the calm beauty of nature.

  - **Do anything with a friend.** Whether you walk, swim, skate, or Zumba, exercising with a friend is more fun and keeps you accountable.

WHAT TO ASK YOUR DOCTOR ABOUT EXERCISE

- How often should I exercise?

- What kind of exercise activity do you recommend?

- I have [name of issue]. What kinds of exercises are best for me?

EAT RIGHT

Food is fuel! But what kind of fuel is best for the multitasking caregiver? The American Heart Association recommends a heart-healthy diet to boost energy and keep you healthy. A heart-healthy diet consists of low sodium, low-fat foods, whole grains, and plenty of fresh fruits and vegetables. Canned or processed foods should be limited since these foods are typically high in sodium or sugar. Controlling portion sizes can reduce caloric intake and overeating. Eating more fruits and vegetables can help keep you full, so you're not as drawn to high-calorie foods and snacks.

A few more suggestions include:

- Plan and prep meals in advance to save time and help you manage your nutrition.

- Keep fresh fruit and vegetables washed and cut up in the refrigerator, ready to eat.

- Portion trail mix or nuts in resealable bags for easy access.

- Increase your water intake and save soft drinks for special occasions or restaurants.

- Opt for whole grains, such as whole-wheat flour, brown rice, and oatmeal—these are excellent sources of fiber while helping regulate blood pressure.

- Enjoy low-fat proteins, such as poultry, fish, lean meat, low-fat dairy products, and eggs.

- Don't forget about legumes, such as beans, lentils, and peas. These are plant-based protein sources that can reduce your cholesterol and fat intake while increasing fiber in your diet.

HOW TO EAT RIGHT

Log your food intake. If nutrition is an issue for you, apps can help track your eating habits and nutrition. Most of these apps have a community feature that allows you to connect with other people to keep you motivated and accountable.

Hydrate. Drink plenty of water or seltzer to stay hydrated and energized. Add sliced fruit, such as lemon or orange slices, to give your water a fresh flavor. Have fun trying new combinations, such as cucumber and lemon or fresh mint leaves.

Rethink your beverage choices. Whenever possible, opt for reduced-sugar or sugar-free drinks. Processed juice, soft drinks, and energy and sports drinks contain lots of added sugars. Even some drinks with "water" in the name have added sugar!

Scour the internet. There is no shortage of healthy recipes, whether your goal is quick-and-easy, low-carb, high-protein, vegetarian, vegan, gluten-free, diabetic—you could find a new recipe for every day. If you're a fan of a paper cookbook, there are countless choices online!

WHAT TO ASK YOUR DOCTOR

- What kind of diet would be best for my health?

- Are there any foods I should avoid?

WHAT TO DO TO STAY CONNECTED

Greet the world. Eye contact and a simple hello can go a long way to establishing first contact. Even if it is a stranger you are passing in the street, say hello and smile. Build new connections by making a habit of greeting every person. That person could become a friend one day and help you when you need it most.

Try something new. Relationships are formed by building memories together. Create unique moments and try new activities with friends and family.

STAY CONNECTED

Caregiving can feel lonely and isolating at times. Juggling a busy schedule of work and caregiving can leave little room for anything else. It can be easy to create a silo where it is just you and your loved one. While socializing with your loved one is important, it is equally vital to connect with other people. Humans are social creatures who seek meaningful relationships. By developing these relationships, you'll build the support team both you and your loved one can depend on.

Yes, staying connected can be challenging. You have to actively work on it instead of expecting others to always come to you. Reach out, and reach out often. Invite a friend over for tea. Chat with people at the park while you and your loved one are out for a walk. Schedule a weekly family dinner or join a social media group. Whatever method you use to connect, when you find a satisfying connection, do it regularly. Bonds between people can only deepen through frequent contact.

HOW TO JOIN A SUPPORT GROUP

Find the best fit. Not all support groups are created equal. Don't be afraid to scout several support groups until you find the one that feels right.

Engage in conversation. To get the most benefit from the group, join the conversation and share what you feel comfortable with. Get to know the people and find those with whom you share a mutual connection.

WHAT TO ASK YOUR SUPPORT GROUP

- Hello, I'm new to this group. What do you recommend for [name of issue]?

- I am struggling with a challenge at home. Can you help me?

- Do you mind sharing your resources for [name of service]?

- I can see that is a difficult situation for you. I understand how you feel. Can I make a suggestion?

- What activities does this support group plan for its participants?

- Would anybody like to participate in a potluck for the next meeting?

SUPPORT GROUPS

Support groups create natural bonds between people who have shared experiences, and are an excellent resource for obtaining advice, expressing frustrations, and offering solutions. Some support groups may schedule fun activities for their members.

Support groups run the gamut from stroke support groups to caregiver support groups and aphasia support groups, to name just a few. Participants may include stroke survivors, caregivers, and/or healthcare professionals. Even if you and your loved one already participate in a stroke support group, consider joining a caregiver support group for yourself. Other caregivers can reduce your stress by expanding your knowledge, recommending resources, or even soothing your worries.

Start your search for a stroke support group using the American Stroke Association's Stroke Support Group Finder located in the Caregivers resources section (page 157). For caregiver support groups, do an internet search of "caregiver support groups near me." You can also subscribe to the Family Caregiver Alliance's Caregiver Online Support Group website, also located in the Caregivers resources section.

BE KIND TO YOURSELF

Being kind to yourself starts by identifying your personal barriers. Ask yourself: *What's getting in my way*? Is it difficult for you to ask for help? Do you feel selfish or guilty when you put your needs first? Maybe you feel a strong responsibility to take care of your loved one that doesn't seem to allow time for you. Think about what gets in the way of taking care of yourself. Identifying thoughts and emotions that increase your stress is the first step to removing personal barriers.

To work through your personal barriers, you may need to really examine your reactions and the emotions behind them. Take your time to understand how you are feeling and why. Writing down your thoughts can help you process them. Confiding in a trusted advisor can help you identify your barriers and ways to help you move forward.

Self-compassion is essential to self-care. Separate yourself from your own self-criticism and give yourself credit for managing the complex tasks of caregiving. Treat yourself the way you would a good friend. Taking care of someone's needs is hard, and you can only do it if you give yourself permission to take care of yourself.

HOW ARE YOU DOING?

If an oxygen mask drops in front of us on an airplane, we are told to put our mask on first before assisting the person next to us. You need to make sure you can breathe so you can assist others. Similarly, we can

WHAT TO DO FOR YOURSELF

Keep your medical and dental appointments. As much as you keep track of your loved one's doctor appointments, don't forget yours, either. Regular checkups are important for maintaining your overall health and wellness.

Celebrate your successes. Celebrate your accomplishments, no matter how small. Treat yourself to a latte at the coffee shop, sing at the top of your lungs in the car, or perform a wild celebratory dance in your living room. Recognize the good things you've done. You deserve it!

WHAT TO ASK YOURSELF

- What brings me joy? How do I incorporate that into my life?

- How did I take care of myself today?

- What made today a good day?

only help our loved ones if we take care of ourselves first. Meet your needs so you can better care for your loved one.

My last piece of advice on self-care is to get plenty of rest. If you can, when the opportunity presents itself, take a 20-minute power nap. Recharge your body and reboot your brain to free it from stress. Are you waiting for your loved one at their physical therapy session? Consider going to the car for a quick nap. Set a timer and get comfortable. Close your eyes, take a deep breath, and relax your body. After a short snooze, you may be surprised how refreshed you feel.

I've talked a lot in this book about how to care for your loved one. Most of the advice I've provided on caring for your loved one can apply to your own self-care. Eat well, exercise regularly, rest up, and connect with others. Live well, laugh loudly, and love wholeheartedly. The caregiver journey is long and challenging, but extremely rewarding. I thank you for allowing me to share this journey with you.

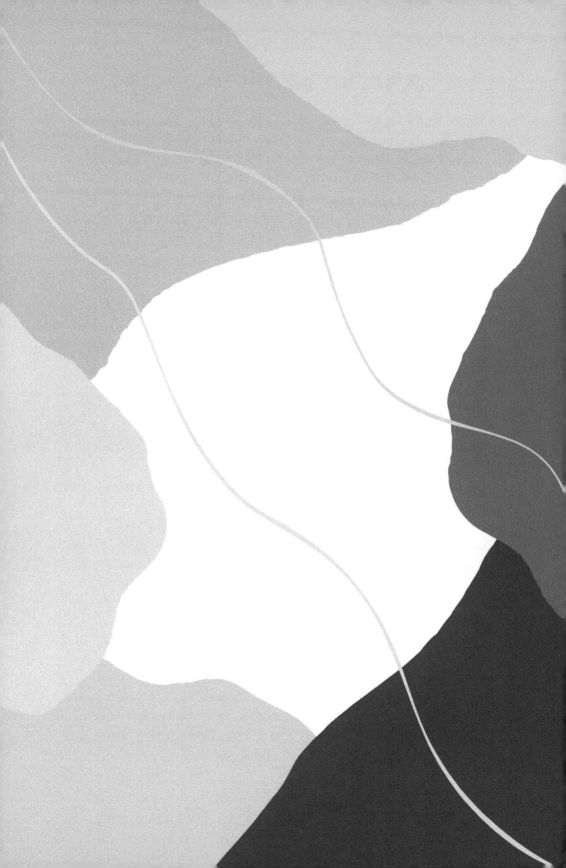

RESOURCES

GENERAL INFORMATION: STROKE

American Stroke Association: Stroke.org

Brain Aneurysm Foundation: BAFound.org

Brain Attack: BrainAttackCoalition.org

National Aphasia Association: Aphasia.org

The Stroke Recovery Foundation: StrokeRecoveryFoundation.org

FOR CAREGIVERS

Daily Caring: DailyCaring.com

Family Caregiver Alliance: Caregiver.org

Family and Medical Leave Act (FMLA): DOL.gov/agencies/whd/fmla

Finance: Caregiver.org/resource/what-every-caregiver-needs
-know-about-money

Hiring In-Home Help: Caregiver.org/resource/hiring-home-help

Legal Planning: Caregiver.org/resource/legal-planning-incapacity

Services by State: Caregiver.org/connecting-caregivers/services-by
-state/?state=national

Today's Caregiver Magazine: Caregiver.com

Well Spouse Association: WellSpouse.org

COMMUNICATION

Amy Speech & Language Therapy Inc.: AmySpeechLanguageTherapy
.com/communication-boards.html

Lingraphica: Aphasia.com/free-communication-boards

National Aphasia Association: Aphasia.org

Say it With Symbols: SayItWithSymbols.com

Wong-Baker FACES Foundation: WongBakerFACES.org

FINANCES

American Heart/American Stroke Association Finances after
Stroke Guide: Stroke.org/en/life-after-stroke/recovery
/managing-your-stroke/finances-insurance-and-assistance

Consumer Financial Protection Bureau—Managing Someone
Else's Money: ConsumerFinance.gov/consumer-tools/managing
-someone-elses-money

Disability Benefits Center: DisabilityBenefitsCenter.org/blog
/stroke-social-security-benefits

National Council on Aging Benefits Checkup: BenefitsCheckup.org

Patient Advocate Foundation: PatientAdvocate.org

Social Security Disability Insurance (SSDI): SSA.gov/benefits/disability

Supplemental Security Income (SSI) Benefits: SSA.gov/benefits/ssi

US Department of Justice—Fraud and Financial Abuse: OJP.gov
/feature/elder-abuse/overview

GOVERNMENT ASSISTANCE

Eldercare Locator: Eldercare.acl.gov

Family and Medical Leave Act: DOL.gov/agencies/whd/fmla

Federal resources for caregivers: USA.gov/disability-caregiver

INSURANCE

Apply for Medicaid: USA.gov/medicaid

Apply for Medicare: SSA.gov/benefits/medicare

Medicaid: Medicaid.gov

Medicare: Medicare.gov

Medicare Supplemental Insurance (Medigap): Medicare
.gov/supplements-other-insurance/whats-medicare
-supplement-insurance-medigap

What Medicare covers: Medicare.gov/what-medicare-covers
/your-medicare-coverage-choices

LONG-TERM CARE RESOURCES

National Adult Day Services Association: NADSA.org

National Respite Network and Resource Center: ArchRespite.org

LEGAL RESOURCES

Advance Directive forms by state: AARP.org/caregiving/financial-legal
/free-printable-advance-directives

Directory of POLST programs: POLST.org/state-programs

National Academy of Elder Law Attorneys: NAELA.org

National Elder Law Foundation: NELF.org

Nolo (legal help website): NOLO.com

MEDICATION ASSISTANCE PROGRAMS

America's Pharmacy: AmericasPharmacy.com

Choice Drug Card: ChoiceDrugCard.com

Familywize Prescription Discount Card: FamilyWize.org/aha

NeedyMeds: NeedyMeds.org/pap

Partnership for Prescription Assistance (PPA) Medicine Assistance Tool: MedicineAssistanceTool.org

RxAssist: RXAssist.org

State pharmaceutical assistance programs (SPAP): StateRXPlans.us /index.php

MENTAL HEALTH RESOURCES

Anxiety and Depression Association of America: ADAA.org

National Helpline Database: VeryWellMind.com/national-helpline-database-4799696

National Institute of Mental Health: NIMH.nih.gov/index.shtml

National Suicide Prevention Lifeline: 1-800-273-TALK (8255)

NUTRITION

The International Dysphagia Diet Standardisation Initiative (IDDSI) Framework: IDDSI.org/Framework

The International Dysphagia Diet Standardisation Initiative (IDDSI) Complete Framework and Detailed Definitions (July 2019): IDDSI.org/IDDSI/media/images/Complete_IDDSI_Framework_ Final_31July2019.pdf

Meals on Wheels America: MealsOnWheelsAmerica.org

REHABILITATION

Commission on the Accreditation of Rehabilitation Facilities: CARF.org

Flint Rehab Stroke Blog: FlintRehab.com/category/stroke

RELAXATION

14 Practical Ways to Relieve Caregiver Stress: DailyCaring.com /14-practical-ways-to-relieve-caregiver-stress/

Relaxation Techniques for Stress Relief: HelpGuide.org/articles/stress /relaxation-techniques-for-stress-relief.htm

A Yoga Sequence for Resilience (Especially for Caregivers): YogaJournal .com/practice/sequence-for-resilience-and-caregivers

RETURN TO WORK

AbilityJOBS (job site for people with disabilities): AbilityJobs.com

American Stroke Association: Return to Work Resources: Stroke.org /en/life-after-stroke/recovery/return-to-work

Job Accommodation Network: AskJAN.org

Office of Disability Employment Policy: DOL.gov/agencies/odep/topics

SAFETY AT HOME

American Stroke Association: Home Modifications: Stroke.org/en/life-after-stroke/recovery/home-modifications

Flint Rehab: 15 Home Modifications for Stroke Patients to Improve Safety: FlintRehab.com/home-modifications-for-stroke-patients

SUPPORT GROUPS

American Stroke Association: Stroke Support Group Finder: Stroke.org/en/stroke-support-group-finder

Family Caregiver Alliance: Support Groups: Caregiver.org/connecting-caregivers/support-groups/

VETERANS' SERVICES

Geriatrics and Extended Care: VA.gov/GERIATRICS

Military Benefits: Benefits.gov/categories/Military%3A%20Active%20Duty%20and%20Veterans

US Department of Veterans Affairs: VA.gov

VA Caregiver Support: Caregiver.va.gov

REFERENCES

"Adapting the Home after a Stroke." The Internet Stroke Center. Accessed February 20, 2021. strokecenter.org/patients /caregiver-and-patient-resources/home-modification/adapting -the-home-after-a-stroke.

"Advance Health Care Directives and POLST." Family Caregiver Alliance. Accessed February 27, 2021. caregiver.org/resource /advance-health-care-directives-and-polst/?via=caregiver -resources,caring-for-another,advanced-illness-and-end-of-life.

"Aphasia." American Speech-Language-Hearing Association. Accessed February 8, 2021. asha.org/practice-portal/clinical-topics/aphasia.

Appelros, Peter. "Prevalence and Predictors of Pain and Fatigue after Stroke: A Population-Based Study." *International Journal of Rehabilitation and Research* 29, no. 4 (December 2006): 329–333.

Boogaard, Kat. "16 Questions You Never Even Realized You Had about Short-Term Disability Benefits." Accessed February 27, 2021. themuse.com/advice/what-to-know-about-short-term-disability.

Bowry, Ritvij, Digvijaya D. Navalkele, and Nicole R. Gonzales. "Blood Pressure Management in Stroke." *Neurology Clinical Practice* 4, no. 5 (October 2014): 419–426.

Bridgeway. "Elder Care Attorneys: 7 Questions to Ask Before You Hire One." August 2, 2019. bridgewayseniorliving.com/elder -care-attorneys-7-questions-to-ask-before-you-hire-one.

Brittain, K. R., S. M. Peet, and C. M. Castleden. "Stroke and Incontinence." *Stroke* 29 (February 1998): 524–528.

"Caregiver Depression: A Silent Health Crisis." Family Caregiver Alliance. 2002. caregiver.org/resource/caregiver-depression -silent-health-crisis.

"Caregiver Statistics: Demographics." Family Caregiver Alliance. April 17, 2019. caregiver.org/caregiver-statistics-demographics.

"Caregiver Statistics: Work and Caregiving." Family Caregiver
Alliance. 2016. caregiver.org/resource/caregiver-statistics
-work-and-caregiving.

"Caregiving." National Institute on Aging. Accessed January 27, 2021.
nia.nih.gov/health/caregiving.

"Caregiving Issues and Strategies." Family Caregiver Alliance. Accessed
January 28, 2021. caregiver.org/caregiving-issues-and-strategies.

"Caring for Adults with Cognitive and Memory Impairment." Family
Caregiver Alliance. Accessed February 8, 2021. caregiver.org
/caring-adults-cognitive-and-memory-impairment.

Carlson, Deirdre. "A Clinical Dietitian's Guide to IDDSI." August 28, 2018.
dietitiansondemand.com/a-clinical-dietitians-guide-to-iddsi.

Chun, Ho-Yan Yvonne, William N. Whitely, Martin S. Dennis, Gillian E.
Mead, and Alan J. Carson. "Anxiety after Stroke." *Stroke* 49
(February 2018): 556–564.

"Communicating with Your Doctor." Family Caregiver Alliance.
Accessed February 18, 2021. caregiver.org/resource
/communicating-your-doctor.

"Communication Tips for Caregivers." American Heart Association.
Accessed January 30, 2021. heart.org/en/health-topics
/caregiver-support/communication-tips-for-caregivers.

"Complete DDSI Framework Detailed Definitions 2.0." International
Dysphagia Diet Standardisation Initiative. July 2019. iddsi.org
/IDDSI/media/images/Complete_IDDSI_Framework_Final
_31July2019.pdf .

"Eating Well after a Stroke." Cleveland Clinic. July 11, 2018.
my.clevelandclinic.org/health/articles/13486-eating-well-after
-a-stroke.

"Exercise Recommendations after Stroke." American Stroke
Association. Accessed February 21, 2021. stroke.org/en
/professionals/stroke-resource-library/post-stroke-care
/patient-focused-rehab-resources/exercise-recommendations
-after-stroke.

"Finances, Insurance and What You Need to Know Post-Stroke."
American Stroke Association. Accessed February 23, 2021.
stroke.org/en/life-after-stroke/recovery/managing-your-stroke
/finances-insurance-and-assistance.

"Financial Planning." Christopher & Dana Reeve Foundation. Accessed
February 23, 2021. christopherreeve.org/living-with-paralysis
/costs-and-insurance/financial-planning.

"Finding the Right Long-Term Care for Your Loved One." AARP.
Accessed March 3, 2021. aarp.org/caregiving/basics/info-2020
/long-term-care.html.

"5 Techniques That Quickly Relieve Caregiver Anxiety." Daily Caring.
Accessed March 7, 2021. dailycaring.com/5-techniques-that-quickly
-relieve-caregiver-anxiety.

Flach, Clare, Walter Muruet, Charles D. A. Wolfe, Ajay Bhalla, and Abdel
Douiri. "Risk and Secondary Prevention of Stroke Recurrence."
Stroke 51 (2020): 2435–2444.

"Grief and Loss." Family Caregiver Alliance. October 2013. caregiver
.org/resource/grief-and-loss.

Hinkle, Janice L., et al. "Poststroke Fatigue: Emerging Evidence and
Approaches to Management: A Scientific Statement for Healthcare
Professionals from the American Heart Association." *Stroke* 48
(May 2017): e159–e170.

"Hiring In-Home Help." Family Caregiver Alliance. Accessed February 3,
2021. caregiver.org/resource/hiring-home-help.

Home Care Assistance. "Sixteen Successful Long-Distance Caregiving
Strategies." Accessed January 27, 2021. homecareassistance.com
/blog/16-successful-long-distance-caregiving-strategies.

"Hope: The Stroke Recovery Guide." American Stroke Association.
December 2020. stroke.org/-/media/stroke files/life-after-stroke
/asa_hope_stroke_recovery_guide_122020.pdf?la=en.

"Incontinence." American Stroke Association. March 19, 2019. stroke
.org/en/about-stroke/effects-of-stroke/physical-effects-of-stroke
/physical-impact/incontinence.

"Intimacy after Stroke." American Stroke Association. December 3,
2018. stroke.org/en/about-stroke/effects-of-stroke
/emotional-effects-of-stroke/intimacy-after-stroke.

"Legal Planning for Incapacity." Family Caregiver Alliance. Accessed
February 15, 2021. caregiver.org/legal-planning-incapacity.

"Life after Stroke Guide." American Stroke Association. 2019.
stroke.org/-/media/stroke-files/life-after-stroke/life-after
-stroke-guide_7819.pdf?la=en.

"Loss of Appetite Coping Strategies." Life Raft Group. August 28, 2013.
liferaftgroup.org/2013/08/loss-appetite-coping-strategies.

Lyons, Mary, et al. "Oral Care after Stroke: Where Are We Now?"
European Stroke Journal 3, no. 4 (December 2018): 347–354.

Meira, Isabella D'Andrea, Tayla Taynan Romao, Henrique Jannuzzelli
Pires do Prado, Lia Theophilo Kruger, Maria Elisa Paiva Pires, and
Priscila Oliveira da Conceicao. "Ketogenic Diet and Epilepsy: What
We Know So Far." *Frontiers in Neuroscience* 13, no. 5 (January
2019): doi.org/10.3389/fnins.2019.00005.

Moawad, Heidi. "How to Say the Right Thing to a Stroke Survivor."
November 3, 2020. verywellhealth.com/how-to-talk-to-a-stroke
-survivor-3146006.

Myint, P. K., E. F. A. Staufenberg, and K. Sabanathan. "Post-Stroke
Seizure and Post-Stroke Epilepsy." *Postgrad Medical Journal* 82,
no. 971 (September 2006): 568–572.

Paolucci, S., et al. "Early versus Delayed Inpatient Stroke Rehabilitation:
A Matched Comparison Conducted in Italy." *Archives of Physical
Medicine and Rehabilitation* 81, no. 6 (June 2000): 695–700.

"Patient Compliance and Solutions." American Stroke Association.
December 6, 2018. stroke.org/en/life-after-stroke/recovery
/managing-your-stroke/compliance-and-solutions.

"PEG Tube Insertion—Discharge." Medline Plus. July 13, 2019. medlineplus.gov/ency/patientinstructions/000900.htm.

"Post Stroke Mood Disorders." American Stroke Association. Accessed February 5, 2021. stroke.org/en/about-stroke/effects-of-stroke /emotional-effects of-stroke/post-stroke-mood-disorders.

Powers, William J., et al. "Guidelines for the Early Management of Patients with Acute Ischemic Stroke: 2019 Update to the 2018 Guidelines for the Early Management of Acute Ischemic Stroke: A Guideline for Healthcare Professionals from the American Heart Association/American Stroke." *Stroke* 50 (Oct 2019): e344–e418.

"Return to Work." American Stroke Association. Accessed February 19, 2021. stroke.org/en/life-after-stroke/recovery/return-to-work.

Rosenblatt, Bob, and Carol Van Steenberg. "Handbook for Long-Distance Caregivers." Family Caregiver Alliance. 2014. caregiver.org/handbook-long-distance-caregivers.

Sanner, Jennifer, et al. "Abstract NS7: Identifying and Understanding Factors Associated with Post-Stroke Anxiety." *Stroke* 50 (January 2019): ANS7.

Saunders, David H., Carolyn A. Greig, and Gillian E. Mead. "Physical Activity and Exercise after Stroke." *Stroke* 45 (November 2014): 3741–3747.

Saver, Jeffrey L. "Time is Brain—Quantified." *Stroke* 37 (January 2006): 263–266.

Schulz, Richard, and Paula R. Sherwood. "Physical and Mental Health Effects of Family Caregiving." *American Journal of Nursing* 108, no. 9 (September 2008): S27.

"Seizure First Aid." Centers for Disease Control and Prevention. September 30, 2020. cdc.gov/epilepsy/about/first-aid.htm.

Semplicini, Andrea, and Lorenzo Calo. "Administering Antihypertensive Drugs after Acute Ischemic Stroke: Timing is Everything." *Canadian Medical Association Journal* 172, no. 5 (March 2005): 625–626.

"Stroke and African Americans." US Department of Health and Human
    Services Office of Minority Health. Accessed January 22, 2021.
    minorityhealth.hhs.gov/omh/browse.aspx?lvl=4&lvlid=28#:~:text
    =African%20Americans%20are%2050%20percent,compared
    %20to%20non%2DHispanic%20whites.

Stroke Association UK. "Pain after Stroke." Accessed February 12, 2021.
    stroke.org.uk/effects-of-stroke/physical-effects-stroke/pain
    -after-stroke.

"Stroke Facts." September 8, 2020. cdc.gov/stroke/facts.htm

"Stroke Pain." Stanford Health Care. Accessed February 12, 2021.
    stanfordhealthcare.org/medical-conditions/brain-and-nerves
    /chronic-pain/types/stroke-pain.html.

Taylor, Jill B. *My Stroke of Insight: A Brain Scientist's Personal Journey.*
    New York: Penguin Group Inc., 2006.

"Thirteen Things Every Stroke Survivor Wished You Knew." Flint
    Rehab. March 20, 2020. flintrehab.com/what-every-stroke-survivor
    -wished-you-knew.

"Thirteen Ways to Improve Your Communication Skills." Elizz. Accessed
    January 29, 2021. elizz.com/caregiver-resources/13-ways-to
    -improve-your-caregiver-communicationskill.

Towfighi, Amytis, et al. "Poststroke Depression: A Scientific Statement
    for Healthcare Professionals from the American Heart Associa-
    tion/American Stroke Association." *Stroke* 48 (December 2016):
    e30–e43.

Treister, Andrew K., Maya N. Hatch, Steven C. Cramer, and Eric Y. Chang.
    "Demystifying Post-Stroke Pain: From Etiology to Treatment." *Physi-
    cal Medicine and Rehabilitation* 9, no. 1 (January 2017): 63–75.

"21 Useful Stroke Exercises to Improve Mobility and Function at Home."
    Flint Rehab. January 13, 2020. flintrehab.com/stroke-exercises.

"What Every Caregiver Needs to Know about Money." Family Caregiver
    Alliance. Accessed February 21, 2021. caregiver.org/resource
    /what-every-caregiver-needs-know-about-money.

"What You Should Know about Post-Stroke Seizures." Healthline. Accessed February 12, 2021. healthline.com/health/stroke /seizure-after-stroke.

"Wills, Trusts and Probate." Nolo. Accessed February 27, 2021. nolo.com /legal-encyclopedia/wills-trusts-estates.

Witkin, Georgia. "6 Ways to Manage Multiple Emotions." April 19, 2019. psychologytoday.com/us/blog/the-chronicles-infertility/201904 /6-ways-manage-multiple-emotions.

INDEX

ACKNOWLEDGMENTS

This book would not have been possible without the love and support of my husband, Brian. He patiently listened to me talk out my ideas, encouraged me when I stared blankly at my computer, not knowing what to write, and quietly reminded me that I needed to take care of myself, too. I am grateful for my personal cheering squad, my kids Lizbeth and Aidan, whose endless hugs kept me motivated.

To my best friend, Latisse Perez, who never hesitates to support me.

Thank you to my friends and colleagues, Leanna Centeno, RN; Gloria Hayman, RN; and Ciarra Rheott, for their unending support. Dan Miulli, DO, FACOS; Heba Fakhoury, DPT; and LeeMae Apacible, RN—your expertise has been invaluable.

Special thanks to my colleague, C.B., who helped proofread my drafts and whose insights were immeasurable.

Thank you to the team at Callisto Media for giving me the opportunity to share my thoughts and positively impact my patients and their families.

To Marie Bartoletti, your perseverance is a model of triumph.

Finally, I would like to extend my gratitude to Alahe Moslemi, my favorite stroke survivor, who never hesitates to support me. It is a pleasure to be a part of your journey.

ABOUT THE AUTHOR

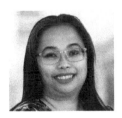

Lucille Jorgensen, RN has been a registered nurse for more than 18 years. Her experience includes telemetry, intensive care, cardiac catheterization, acute rehabilitation, quality management, and patient safety. Lucille is certified in Lean Healthcare and is a TeamSTEPPS Master Trainer. She developed a passion for stroke care while serving as a certified stroke program coordinator for a large academic hospital in Southern California.

Outside of work, Lucille is happily married with two kids. She has served as a Girl Scout leader for nine years and an active Cub Scout and Boy Scout volunteer for seven years. She is an avid reader, movie buff, foodie, and really big convention-going nerd/geek.

CPSIA information can be obtained
at www.ICGtesting.com
Printed in the USA
BVHW022207200122
626712BV00008B/43